The Adventures of
CADET CODY

The True Story of How One Family and Their Pet Dog Survived R-Day, Beast, and Plebe Year at West Point

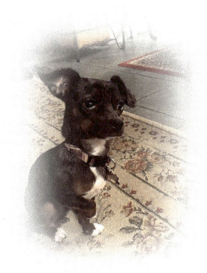

JOSEPH E. OLSAVSKY

PAGE PUBLISHING, INC.
Conneaut Lake, PA

First originally published by Page Publishing 2021

The contents of this book, *The Adventures of Cadet Cody: The True Story of How One Family and Their Pet Dog Survived R-Day, Beast, and Plebe Year at West Point*, was privately produced and are not endorsed by or to be considered as official views of the United States Military Academy at West Point, New York, US Service Academies, United States Army, US Department of Defense, or West Point Associate of Graduates.

All names used are real; no fictitious names are reflected in the book. To protect privacy, in certain instances, individual's titles are used rather than first and last names.

Unless otherwise acknowledged by the citations listed in the Notes section, which reflect sources of certain excerpts captured in the book, all writing was done by Joseph E. and Cathy D. Olsavsky, parents of USMA Cadet Nathaniel J. Olsavsky, Class of 2021.

ISBN 978-1-6624-3682-6 (pbk)
ISBN 978-1-6624-3683-3 (digital)

Printed in the United States of America

Dear family,

You were the inspiration that started this adventurous journey along with our very first family pet, Cody. We became closer through Cadet Cody and even more so with each passing day. And to our adventurer, Cody, you will always be our lil' buddy.

Love,
Dad

CONTENTS

PREFACE

WHAT IS IT about certain times in our lives that make them stand out from the others? Many of us can still remember the time when TV stations signed off to end a night. After midnight, the majority of broadcasters in both Canada and the United States turned off their transmitters and went off the air. This act of signing off was often celebrated with patriotic fanfare, firstly with a station identification, then the playing of the national anthem, and ending with a stirring short film.

I was born in 1964 and vaguely recalled watching a movie clip of a US Air Force jet flying high in the clouds as the words of one of the most enduring aviation poems was read to end the night: "High Flight" by John Gillespie Magee.

> *Oh! I have slipped the surly bonds of Earth*
> *And danced the skies on laughter-silvered wings;*
> *Sunward I've climbed, and joined the tumbling mirth*
> *Of sun-split clouds—and done a hundred things*
> *You have not dreamed of—wheeled and soared and swung*
> *High in the sunlit silence. Hov'ring there,*
> *I've chased the shouting wind along, and flung*
> *My eager craft through footless halls of air...*

Up, up the long, delirious burning blue
I've topped the wind-swept heights with easy grace
Where never lark, or ever eagle flew—
And, while with silent, lifting mind I've trod
The high untrespassed sanctity of space,
Put out my hand, and touched the face of God.

My father loved that poem. He was a deeply patriotic man—a man of faith and a true family man. Ignatius (Iggy) J. Olsavsky worked in the coal mines of southwestern Pennsylvania for thirty-three years and saw that my brothers and sisters and I were not without; we were provided for. He saw to it, and my mom saw to it. We didn't have much, but we had it all.

Both my mom and dad loved to read, and yes, they could write as well. Mom's cursive looked as if it was eloquently chiseled by an angel—exquisite, expressive, and harmoniously beautiful. However, Dad's penmanship had something to be desired, and let's just say this apple didn't fall far from the tree.

I remember my parents anxiously waiting for the mailman to deliver a letter from my older brother, Ed, who enlisted in the United States Coast Guard in the early '70s. Ed found himself stationed in the Aleutian Islands, Alaska, and then Yap, an island group located in the western Pacific Ocean. Words can't describe the sight of them seeing a letter postmarked from a place far and away. They had that very same look when, ten years later, my brother Tom enlisted in the United States Army Reserves.

The kitchen table served as their joint writing desk on many afternoons and evenings, two cups of coffee always nearby, along with pen and paper in hand. They would compose letters only a parent could write—words known but to them, Ed and Tom alone. They would beam with joy and pride knowing that their sons willingly and selflessly volunteered to join a unique group, who, like so many others before them, made the choice to step up to honor, support, and defend our country.

Reading and writing were a mainstay for Mom and Dad. It was rare not to see them with a book in their hands when they finally found some spare time. Following the passing of my mom in 1995, then my dad in 1998, my brothers and sisters were pleasantly surprised to discover our father's affection for writing—pen, paper, and story writing. Tucked away, handwritten on now time-weathered paper, was an unfinished story: *The Mushroom That Covered Pennsylvania*. My five sisters and four brothers, or the ten little Indians as Dad referred to us, couldn't help but smile when we found his story stashed with his personal paperwork.

Now some two decades-plus later, my thoughts often turn to the what-ifs. What if Mom and Dad were still alive today? The joy they would have felt seeing me walking Hillary, our daughter, down the aisle on her wedding day. The compassion, love, and prayers they would have given Sam, our youngest son when he underwent spinal fusion surgery. And the delight and pride seeing their grandson Nate, our middle child, receiving an appointment to the United States Military Academy at West Point seventy-two years after Dad hung up his Army uniform upon World War II coming to an end.

If these two time-honored nonagenarians were alive today, I'm certain they would be sitting at the kitchen table, with pen and paper clasped between feeble arthritic fingers, writing away.

ACKNOWLEDGMENTS

THE COMPLETION OF this book, my first attempt at finding the discipline and wherewithal to compose the thoughts running wild in my mind, would not have been possible without Cathy, my wonderful wife and best friend. You spent countless hours reading and commenting on the pages as they materialized. Without your unconditional support, love and thoughtfulness, this book would have never come to be.

Thank you Sam, Hillary and Nate for inspiring me. And simply being more than loving children. You are what makes the world go round. I love you more than what any words can describe.

To my sister Susie and brother-in-law, Jim, you have been our friends and confidantes. Thank you for joining us along this West Point journey and sharing our memories. I would be remiss; however, if I did not mention that I am still at a loss as to how Susie and Cathy thought this was going to be a children's book. You never know. Maybe I will take another go at being creative and give writing another try.

A special thank you to all the young men and women we encountered and came to know through our very own West Point Cadet, Nate. Your selfless commitment to Duty, Honor and Country is comforting and touches our hearts. Our great nation, these United States of America are in the best of hands. May God continue to bless and watch over you.

To Diana and Kendall, the page design coordinators, and cover page artists at Page Publishing. You have been extremely helpful and brought a lifelong dream of mine to fruition.

Lastly, a special thank you to Cody, our Lil Buddy. I love ya! After all these years, who would have thought that such a tiny canine bundle would have been the secret to tearing down my reluctance for a family pet. You opened a new world to me!

CHAPTER 1

Placed on a Collision Course

WELCOME TO OUR story. Or, as you will see, it is more of a story within a story. *The Adventures of Cadet Cody* covers the send-off and goodbye to our soon-to-be West Point cadet. During this time and through his six weeks of cadet basic training at the United States Military Academy, with no direct contact to the outside world, we find comfort and an outlet to deal with our separation. An energetic, loving bundle of canine joy comes to the rescue. The newest addition to our family, Cody, a warm, sleek cocker spaniel mix, forms the genesis for Cadet Cody.

The Adventures of Cadet Cody story comes to life in the summer weeks of July and August 2017 during the exchange of letters to our Plebe, Nate. Heartfelt and separated by time and distance, we revert to the antiquated pastime of writing letters, pen and paper in hand. Our imagination, Cody's antics, our family experiences, and activities come to life in a cartoon, storylike fashion.

These tales speak to our very first visit and impressions of West Point. Intimidating, prisonlike, it leaves you with a Harry Potter, Hogwarts-type of feeling and mindset. These emotions and visions soon change as if a veil of fog is lifted, showing the incredible beauty, respect, and hallowed appreciation of one of the oldest military service academies in the world. We hope you enjoy our stories and what is to come. All true. All from the heart.

The United States Military Academy, better known as West Point, is perhaps one of the best and most prestigious military academies in the world. West Point is among a renowned cache of military institutes that include as follows:

- United States Naval Academy, Annapolis, Maryland, USA
- The Royal Military Academy, Sandhurst, Camberley, United Kingdom
- The Special Military School of Saint Cyr, Coëtquidan, France
- PLA National Defense University, Beijing, China
- General Staff Academy, Moscow, Russia, and
- The National Defense Academy of Japan, Yokosuka, Japan

Formally established in 1802, West Point is located on the scenic Hudson River in New York and was identified by General George Washington as the most strategic position in America during the American Revolution. *"The establishment of a military academy, upon a respectable and extensive basis, has ever been considered by me to be an object of the highest national importance."* General Washington's words on December 12, 1799, laid this foundation. Today, West Point has the distinction of being the longest continuously occupied United States military installation.

Those cadets who pass through the historic and time-honored institution affectionately find themselves as the next link in the Long Gray Line. The Long Gray Line reflects the gray cadet uniforms and the exceptional young men and women who experience the wool fabric, stiff collars, and other pageantry among the many uniforms worn throughout their time training to be United States Army officers.

In his farewell speech given to the Corps of Cadets at West Point on May 12, 1962, General Douglas MacArthur tells the corps that *"your guide posts stand out like a tenfold beacon in the night: duty, honor, country… The Long Gray Line has never failed us."* These words become a beacon for our family as we move forward and become part of the West Point family of families.

The Adventures of Cadet Cody: The True Story of How One Family and Their Pet Dog Survived R-Day, Beast, and Plebe Year at West Point is our humble and proud emotional journey for our soon-to-be new cadet. A warm, sunny, beautiful Sunday (July 2, 2017) morning departure from our home and loving dog, Cody, and the scenic hills of southwestern Pennsylvania in Somerset County placed us on a collision course with the imminent sixty-second farewell on Reception Day (July 3, 2017) for our Class of 2021 son—Nate.

And this is Nate's first step in a long, difficult, emotional, mental, and physical journey to be next in the Long Gray Line where he and many like him will be standing as shining, piercing lights for this great nation. As an outsider looking in, what an incredible feeling!

In forty-seven months, these cadets will be assigned to one of seventeen Branches of the US Army. Officer Branch Specialties of the Army include Infantry, Air Defense Artillery, Armor, Aviation, Corps of Engineers, and Field Artillery, to name several. Based on an Order of Merit List (OML) system, the cadets will pick the posts they want until the last cadet is left with the final posting on the wall.

Many will find their way to Fort Benning, Georgia; Fort Bliss, Texas; Fort Bragg, North Carolina; or Fort Campbell, Kentucky, as well as overseas posts in Italy, Germany, and South Korea. Interestingly, many Army insiders rank the top five duty stations/posts as

1. Casera-Ederle, Italy
2. Kelley Barracks, Stuttgart, Germany
3. Fort Lewis, Washington
4. Fort Carson, Colorado
5. Yongsan, South Korea

These soon-to-be second lieutenants have eyes wide-open. It's go time!

Nothing can prepare a parent when they hear that their child is joining the military. But you come to a realization that this is a choice they have made and it is their decision. And as parents, we are here to provide our unending love and support. Our child has gone from the young boy playing in the yard, kicking the soccer ball, and making his way through classrooms and, more recently, the halls of high school and through the gates of graduation. Now, oh yes, now a new chapter and journey in his life is underway.

Our son, our new USMA West Point Army cadet, is on an exciting path that will take him to different parts of the world. Nate is in the throes and, hopefully, more so in the midst of greater joys, pleasures, and lifelong experiences and memories with a new extended family and group of friends—his brothers and sisters in arms.

This is one of the many reasons we continue to be increasingly awe inspired with each visit to West Point. Watching these cadets walk in their Army green ACUs, their white-over-grays, and other uniforms brings a warmth to the heart. Our thoughts and prayers grow stronger for all these young men and women, these brave cadets that walk among the serene, calm, and hallowed grounds of West Point.

Sit back and indulge yourself in the epic journey of a young man traveling through what only a select group have experienced. This is our narrative, our story, with the help of Cody as we recount the luster of Reception Day, Beast, Acceptance Day, and Plebe year at West Point.

Enjoy!

CHAPTER 2

The Waiting

"GOOD MORNING, NATE! What time did you get home last night?" Cathy asked.

"It was close to 1:00 AM," Nate said.

"Well, you can sleep in the car. I'm sure Sam will sleep too," Cathy replied.

The drive from scenic Friedens, Pennsylvania (which is about fifteen minutes from the Flight 93 National Memorial), to West Point is about six hours, and now, looking back on this day, we've come to make this car ride many, many times since that R-Day departure from home to the gates of the United States Military Academy.

It is early Sunday morning, 6:00 AM-ish, July 2, 2017, and the sun is shining brightly in the yard, sharp crisp rays penetrating into the kitchen and the grass is still wet with dew, but the humidity is bearable. The blue skies are welcoming, too, as we begin to go through Nate's checklist.

Cathy repeats, "Nate, do you have all your paperwork? Driver's license, passport, immunization record?"

Soon enough, we'll be packing the car. Sam and I are mostly quiet as everyone grabs a light bite to eat for breakfast—a small glass of orange juice, toast, and granola bars. There's a nervousness in the air, not so much of an uneasy, stomach-turning feeling, but more of the heading off into the unknown what will tomorrow and the next day and the next day hold. High school graduation seemed like forever in the past although it was barely a few weeks ago. Gift cards, presents, and remnants of Nate's Somerset Area Senior High School year still filled his bedroom and other parts of the house. Our eighteen-year-old boy! We struggle to think our young boy, what am I saying? Young man, yes, now such a strong, handsome, determined young man who will soon be left to the rigors and devices and overarching discipline of the United States Army.

Oftentimes, Cathy and I look into each other's eyes, and in some strange sort of way, our thoughts seem to be telepathically transmitting. Where did the last eighteen years go? What does the next six weeks hold in store for Nate? How will we get through this emotional roller coaster of separation anxiety during Beast? Soon we'll be passing the gates of West Point and counting down our last sixty seconds before we say goodbye. Next stop, saying hello to the many unknowns of the military way of life for our son—the West Point life!

"Hey, Nate, what did you think when Father O'Neill called you out at four o'clock Mass yesterday?" I asked.

"Pretty neat, I wasn't expecting that," Nate said.

Father Daniel O'Neill was the pastor of St. Peter's Catholic Church in Somerset, Pennsylvania. He had a passion for all sports, and that's putting it mildly. And he was a die-hard Philadelphia Eagles' fan. He breathed everything Eagles. But all of St. Peter's took consolation in knowing that Father O'Neill backed the Pittsburgh Penguins. The Pittsburgh Steelers was his fallback team, and he took every opportunity to insert any and all sports into a mass homily or give the St. Peter's school students an earful of sports trivia.

Both Nate and Sam, really our entire family, became particularly close to Father O'Neill and St. Peter's parish. The boys attended and graduated from St. Peter's school that had enrollment from kindergarten through sixth grade. It wasn't too long ago, over seven years in real time, that Nate graduated from St. Peter's back in 2010. Cathy got him a pendant and chain as a graduation gift—St. Sebastian, the patron saint of soldiers, athletes, and those who desire a saintly death.

Nate loved soccer, Area Youth Soccer Association (AYSO) teams, Western Pennsylvania traveling teams, junior high, and finishing his soccer play in high school. Soccer, soccer, soccer.

Father O'Neill would keep track of Somerset High School sports standings and zing Nate every so often. Hockey became such an easy target during Nate's junior year in high school. The varsity team eventually finished the season with a *defeated* record. Yes, defeated, as in not winning a single game. But there's more to this story and this hockey season. The junior varsity hockey team was placed as the fourth seed in the JV playoff schedule. There was still some hope for Nate and his teammates. Some sort of redemption was possible. And as fate would have it, many of the hockey team players who played on the defeated varsity team saw their way over the next two weeks to raise the championship trophy and claim the Junior Varsity Laurel Mountain Hockey Athletic Conference title. Quite the emotional ride, bottoming out, then rising to the top!

Father O'Neill walked to the podium before beginning 4:00 PM Mass.

He began, "We have a special young man that I would like to call attention to. Nate, can you please stand up? Tomorrow, Nathan Olsavsky will be departing for the United States Military Academy at West Point. I want you to know that we will be thinking about you and praying for your success as you undertake these next steps in service to our country."

Nate was flushed and somewhat teary-eyed, as was Cathy and me. Father O'Neill commended Nate, and his remaining words are still a blur as I softly sobbed. Cathy, Nate, Sam, Hillary, Jacob (our son-in-law), and I were seated in the pews at the front of the church. I remember Nate turning around to face those attending Mass and gently lifting his arm to wave. I think it was a mixed wave, a lift of his arm to say thank you and probably one more so to indicate that he was saying his goodbye. A goodbye to familiarity—Somerset, St. Peter's, friends, a goodbye to so many things that he found comfort and strength in. So many times, we see how objects, decisions, activities from our past come full circle to meet us in present time. This Sunday morning was one of those moments.

Cathy checks in with Nate again. "Nate, do you think you'll be allowed to keep your St. Sebastian chain on during training?"

Nate simply answers, "I'm not sure."

Our family is an indirect military family. Cathy and I were not in the military. My father and grandfather each served in the US Army—my dad in World War II and the Korean War and my grandfather in World War I. Nate's middle name, Joseph, ties back to his paternal great-grandfather, Joseph Liko, who served as a private in the Army during World War I.

Every piece of information that comes our way regarding West Point and the Army is new territory. Cathy and I read about R-Day, or Reception Day. The word *reception* makes it sound like an all-arms-open welcoming, fun-filled, smiles and laughter day camp in the making. But we've seen the YouTube videos of the Cadets in the Red Sash. Nope! West Point shouldn't be mistaken as Camp Fun.

Young men and women are screaming, "New cadet! Step up to my line! Not on my line, not over my line, not behind my line! Step up to my line!" The experienced cadre would say.

Cathy and I have done a lot of *research* on what Nate can expect for this first introduction to West Point known as R-Day. Cathy has *The Mom's Guide to Surviving West Point* by Lisa Browne Joiner and Deborah L. W. Boszel. The West Point Parents' Club of Western Pennsylvania also sent the West Point Parents' Class of 2021 Survival Guide. The guide contains so much information and all great stuff and is tremendously helpful!

- A copy of the 2017–2018 USMA-WP calendar
- The cadet prayer
- Club officers
- Contact information
- Overview of R-Day
- Items needed for R-Day
- Communicating with your cadet
- Acceptance Day weekend
- Cadet life
- And other notable cadet events and tidbits

It seems like we've dotted all the i's and crossed the t's in preparing for this moment, departing home and a certain yet particular way of life—get Nate and Sam off to school, hockey games, soccer games, musical, senior events. Looking back, those now seem somewhat routine, but a comforting routine. No getting around the West Point buildup and pending drama; change is on its way! A new beginning for Nate and a different feeling for Cathy, Sam, and me being down one person at home.

Sam teases with a simultaneous smile and chuckle. "You're going to be bald."

Nate acknowledged Sam's comment quietly and somberly. Easy to see Nate's thoughts are elsewhere. Plus, he sounds a bit stuffy and congested. Oh no! T minus one day until R-Day and the onset of a summer cold. Go figure.

Cathy asks, "Nate, do you want to take some Dayquil or Tylenol Cold and Flu?"

"No," he says. "I'll be fine."

Sam and Nate are probably like so many other brothers—best of friends, ready to antagonize in a heartbeat and visibly connected in their love for each other. This Sunday-morning departure to West Point is just one of the many emotional events our sons have closely shared as brothers.

A quote from an unknown source states, "There's no other love like the love for a brother." These words ring so true.

Year 2017 began with apprehension, uncertainty, and fear. Sam was diagnosed with scoliosis two and a half years earlier and was measured and fitted with a support brace that went from under his arms down through his hips, which he had to wear for about twenty-two hours a day. Even after wearing his brace for about ten months, his orthopedic specialist determined that the curvature in Sam's spine had progressed so rapidly it required surgery. It was time for a surgical correction. On March 29, the procedure was performed at Allegheny Health Network in Pittsburgh, Pennsylvania, where spinal fusion was done. It was about a ten-and-a-half-hour surgery in which they put screws in Sam's vertebrae. He has two eighteen-inch titanium rods running down each side of his spine covered with bone chips, along with several vertebrae fused for support. He was two inches taller after the procedure.

And soon enough, our fifteen-year-old would be posing with the crew of a C-130 Hercules aircraft with *2nd Lt. Samuel Olsavsky* inscribed above the cockpit at the 911th Airlift Wing, Pittsburgh Air Reserve Station.

Sam was nominated by the staff at Allegheny Health Network for the Pilot for a Day Program. On June 27, he was sworn in as an honorary second lieutenant. What an incredible day! You talk about the red carpet being rolled out. Wow. That's exactly what the 911th Airlift Wing did for Sam. From the welcome sign at the entrance of the base, *Welcome, Pilot for a Day Samuel Olsavsky and Family,* to the outpouring of care, support, and genuine love for our son. Thank you just wasn't enough on that day.

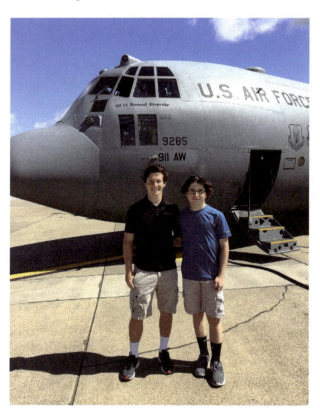

The commander of the 911th Airlift Wing and his crew were quick to give Nate a hard time when they saw his black West Point polo shirt.

"West Point, huh?" one of the flight officers teased Nate.

"Yes, sir," Nate replied. "I report on July 3."

The 911th officers listened attentively as Nate told them how he was nominated for an appointment to the Class of 2021 by Rep. Keith Rothfus of Pennsylvania's twelfth congressional district.

Again, they teased, "You know the Air Force has a nice service academy" as many chuckled. They would then go on to say how Sam beat Nate to his second lieutenant bars. We all smiled!

Nate accompanied Sam during the day's activities. Together they experienced a virtual reality parachute drop, rode in a Humvee, taxied along the tarmac in a carrier jet, saw a taser demo and canine unit, and Sam also received personal dog tags and a wooden replica of a C-130. Sam said the experience was something that will always stay with him.

Quietly, we thought Nate's dog tags will be coming soon enough, ones that will be encircling his neck and dangling like his St. Sebastian medal and chain.

Interestingly enough, another type of canine was part of the New Year. On Saturday, January 28, 2017, Cathy, Nate, Sam, and I welcomed Cody, an eight-week-old, four-pound dark black-brown molted, white-chested and white-tipped-pawed cocker spaniel-Chi-huahua mix.

Sam's spinal fusion was scheduled for March 29, 2017, and Cathy and I discussed how best to handle his recovery. Sam would miss the remainder of the school year which timed perfectly with his last grading period. We worked with the Somerset School Guidance Office, and Sam would be homeschooled two to three times a week when he gained back enough strength. Cody (not yet named), it was decided, would be a warm addition and aid in Sam's recovery. Hillary picked our newest family member up from an Amish breeder in Lancaster, Pennsylvania.

Sam and Nate were clueless on that late January winter Saturday afternoon. They knew absolutely nothing about our plans for a warm, tiny lapdog. That Saturday morning for Sam and Nate was spent at the Somerset High School gym, playing in an indoor soccer tournament, one of countless soccer tournaments our boys would participate in. But this one had a surprising end! We pulled into the driveway at 1:30 PM. A knock at the door. Sam and Nate were curious when Hillary appeared. They wondered why she made the trip from her apartment in Carlisle, Pennsylvania, on this sunny mid-January Saturday afternoon.

In her hands was the tiniest, cutest, and quietly frightened warm bundle of soft fur, staring with large, marble-like eyes. It was a pup! Oh, how cute! How adorable!

Sam asked Hillary, "Hill, did you get another dog?"

Hillary already had her precious Stella, a blue Australian cattle dog. Hillary loved her so much, and Remi, too, Jacob's matching brownish red Australian cattle dog. What a pair.

Hillary replied, "Nope, this puppy is for you!"

Sam's eyes opened wide, and both he and Nate grew smiles like we've never seen before. Surprised doesn't even begin to describe the look on their faces. In a matter of minutes, the newest member of our family had a name—Cody.

I see Sam and Nate exchanging glances on this quiet July Sunday morning. The love for a brother and the love from a brother. Before too long, I imagine that Nate will be experiencing a similar type of feeling for a new brotherhood—his fellow cadets at West Point. These individuals from all walks of life, from all over the United States and other parts of the world will be his new extended family.

Is he ready for this? I think to myself. *What challenges will Nate encounter, what disappointment, and what successes? Is he ready? Absolutely*, I answer myself.

I think about the congressional nomination process and his West Point journey to obtain an appointment. And that's a whole other story. One thing stands out clearly, however: Nate's words in his nomination application letter addressing why he desires to attend the United States Military Academy at West Point.

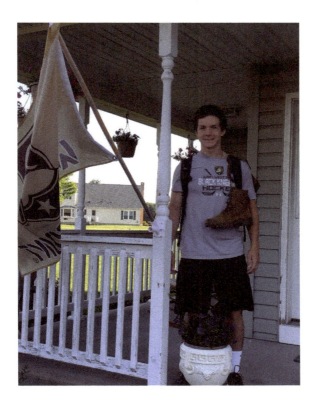

Nate wrote in his personal essay, in part, the following: "A quote from an unknown author states, 'Only two defining forces have ever offered to die for you: Jesus Christ and the American soldier. One died for your soul, the other for your freedom.' I am willing to sign up for the responsibilities that come with being an American soldier."

Again, I think, *Is Nate ready?* I wipe away another tear.

Cathy asks the group, "What do you think? Let's get Nate's stuff packed in the car, and we'll get going."

A few trips from the main entranceway around to the front of the garage and the last of our luggage and Nate's belongings for R-Day are put in place. It's go time!

Well, almost go time. It's photo-op time. Cathy is famous for her front-door photography moments. First day of school, Christmas, Easter, Mother's Day, Father's Day, family vacations—all these events get any and all of us to pose for a picture, either directly from Cathy or timed on the tripod. This picture-perfect, bright, sunny, warm July 2 Sunday morning is no different. Cathy asks Nate to stand with Sam on the porch, in front of the doorway.

Click. Now one with me and Nate. *Click, click.* I take the camera from Cathy and take a few shots of her and Nate. And the last picture is of Nate with his T8 Bifida Army combat boots from US Patriot Tactical tied together and hanging over his shoulder. The final click. We're not sure of when Nate will return back home for that first visit after surviving Beast, and everything else West Point has in store as the end of summer, without fail, will turn to early fall.

"Nate, how do you think Cody will react when he sees you for the first time again when you come back home? Do you think he'll remember you?" asks Sam.

We do a check of our seat belts. All buckled up. Cathy leads us in a calming, reserved prayer, and I back slowly out of our driveway.

Goodbye, Friedens, Pennsylvania. Goodbye, Somerset County. Goodbye, friends and family. Goodbye, Cody. I wonder if these are just a few thoughts racing through Nate's mind as we depart home. The culmination of the previous two-plus years of hard work, dedication, and commitment are here! The next chapter in Nate's West Point saga is underway. This six-hour drive would be our new cadet's path to the scenic Hudson Valley in lower New York State. Nate will soon be walking among the castellated architecture of Washington Hall, Eisenhower (Ike) Hall, Bradley Barracks, the Old Cadet Chapel, and the many other historic buildings and sights that he will call home. This is the United States Military Academy. This is West Point!

The drive along Pennsylvania Routes 219 and 22 going past Altoona up to Interstate 80 are uneventful. We pass State College and Penn State University. Penn State and the University of Pittsburgh were dueling parts of Nate's collegiate backup plan if West Point didn't work out. I-80 eastbound to I-81 meeting up to I-84, we cross the Pennsylvania/New York state line. Our destination is just over one hour away.

"Well, Nate, we're here," says Cathy as we make the turn into the Holiday Inn Express in Fort Montgomery, New York.

It's midafternoon, 4:00 PM. "We can stop at Rite Aid and get you some Tylenol Cold Max," Cathy tells Nate. "Hopefully, that will help alleviate some of your stuffiness and watery eyes."

Sam has already decided what and where we'll have to go for dinner later this evening. An easy decision for him—Tony's Pizza in Highland Falls, New York, a stone's throw outside the security gates to West Point. We've been to Tony's on two previous visits to the academy, and Sam really didn't put the dinner choice up for discussion. Nate, Cathy, and I are fans of Tony's pizza and the antipasti salad, so it's an easy and argue-free selection.

All our luggage and Nate's singular bag, an Eagle Creek pack, are placed inside our hotel room in an orderly way. Everyone is relaxed and stretched out after being in the car. Cathy tells Nate that we'll go through all his paperwork after dinner—immunization records, mileage, hotel receipt for reimbursement, passport, driver's license, etc. We rack our brains for the nth time checking and rechecking Nate's list to make sure we haven't forgotten or misplaced anything. For the next hour, the hotel room is quiet and uneventful, yet there is a level of preoccupation and expectancy. Tomorrow morning will be here before too long.

"Hey, family, what do you say? Are you guys hungry?" I ask the group. "We'll stop at Rite Aid first and get some cold medicine."

Cathy says she's feeling like a cold is coming on too. I park the car and leave her and the boys to relax. In a matter of minutes, I walk back out the front of the store with the blue Tylenol. Both Cathy and Nate take a capful of the blue liquid Tylenol Cold and Flu medicine and chase it with bottled water that we have in the car from the trip today. Hot, humid, and plenty of sunshine as the temperature pushes toward 90°F. I tell Nate I'm sure they'll be pushing all of you (the new cadets, Class of 2021) to drink plenty of water and stay hydrated.

Cathy and I repeat and repeat the same message, "Nate, make sure you drink plenty of water during R-Day processing. It's going to be a long, hot trying day."

Nate looks at us, tacitly responding, "Sure."

His thoughts are elsewhere.

We slowly drive down Main Street in Highland Falls, New York, and easily find a parking spot, a few steps away from Tony's. We get quickly seated at a table but see that other families, other parents with Class of 2021 cadets, have the identical dinner plans. Understandably so. The selection of local restaurants near Highland Falls, West Point, are limited but good—the Park, Schade's, West Point Pizza, American Burrito, Hacienda, Dong Fong, Maria Bonita, Barnstormer's BBQ in Fort Montgomery, and the default McDonald's.

It takes the waitress some time to take our drink orders. The air-conditioning inside the restaurant is struggling to keep up with the outside heat. It is toasty!

I comment, "Maybe we should have ordered take out. Eat back at the hotel."

Sam is unfazed, and he has a high tolerance for extreme weather—hot and cold. It's after 6:00 PM, and both Cathy and Nate are struggling to engage in conversation. Actually, Nate has his eyes closed and is falling asleep in front of us. Cathy says she feels like she could go to sleep too. Perhaps this emotional roller-coaster ride, soon to enter into its next chapter, has caught up to us.

Or maybe there's just a simple logical explanation for their tiredness. Perhaps. We finish eating our pepperoni pizza at Tony's and make our ten-minute drive back to the Holiday Inn Express. I grab my West Point 1802 ball cap and the Tylenol from the car, press Floor 2 on the elevator button, and walk into our room.

"Oh my goodness!" Cathy's voice echoes in the room. She's holding the blue Tylenol bottle and points at the label. "You got Tylenol PM. No wonder Nate and I were falling sleep!"

Sam jokingly says, "Dad, way to go! You drugged Mom and Nate."

I shake my head and unreservedly apologize, "I'm so sorry."

Nate lays out his clothes for Monday morning—lime green Under Armour, Army West Point shirt, tan khaki shorts, boxers, white socks, and his Brooks tennis shoes.

It's only a little after 9:30 PM; we finish brushing our teeth and find our way into bed. The air-conditioning hums in the hotel room, and we hear people walking the hallway. It's been a memorable, emotion-packed, and love-filled day.

"Good night, Nate. Good night, Sam. Love you, sleep tight."

This July 2, Sunday, is drifting away. Nate, Sam, Cathy, and I fall fast asleep.

Beep, beep, beep, beep, beep. Early Monday morning. The 4:45 AM alarm sounds on my iPhone.

I nudge Cathy and ask, "What do you think? Let's wake up Nate. He can hop in the shower first."

Breakfast is light on this early July 3 Monday morning—granola bars, blueberry muffins, and fruit cups. Cathy and I each go for our much-needed cups of coffee. Nate and Sam choose between apple juice and bottled water.

Reception Day, or R-Day, as it is better known, is the beginning of cadet candidate's arrival at the United States Military Academy at West Point. It marks the beginning of their time at the historic institute where these young men and women will undergo a transformation from their civilian status.

And at the end of a long day, with bleachers packed solid of parents, brothers, sisters, etc., they will take their oath on the central cadet parade ground. This open-fielded area, known as the Plain, hosts the largest number of monuments and statues, and inside the stone-walled structures of West Point includes Washington Monument, Thayer Monument, Eisenhower Monument, MacArthur Monument, Kosciuszko Monument, and Sedgwick Monument.

Passing through the guard posts seems different this morning.

West Point has three access points: The Main Thayer Gate, which is located on the west bank of the Hudson River near Buffalo Soldier Field and Stony Lonesome Gate, is open twenty-four hours for visitor's access. The Washington Gate is open every day of the week for Department of Defense (DOD) personnel during certain hours. Thayer Gate will be our entryway for Nate's scheduled—6:20 AM pickup for R-Day Group 2 processing. The approach to the guards is orderly, and the flow of traffic moves quickly along. A brief handoff of our IDs and we are directed to Buffalo Soldier parking lot.

This is it! I park midway down in the lot. The realization of Nate, our beloved son, entering West Point, joining the US Army, committing to place himself in harm's way hits with a wallop. The feelings are somewhere between stage fright and sensory deprivation. I envisage all of us here today are all numb.

The line of other new cadets and their loved ones is probably fifty people in length. Some new cadets are wearing their boots, others, their dress black shoes. And some of the boys, young men rather, are sporting very long full hair.

R-Day arrival processing is scheduled in three-group intervals with multiple shuttles taking everyone to Eisenhower (Ike) Hall. After a short orientation on this already-scorching July Monday, the cadet candidates will have sixty seconds to say goodbye to their families. For the next six weeks, contact with family members, if any, is extremely limited.

Nate, Sam, Cathy, and I slowly move up the line of people as boarding on the shuttle buses continues. One by one, we inch along. Some cadet candidates have boot laces tied and dangling over their shoulders. Many in the crowd are carrying cups of coffee. And with the temperatures rising, many moms are pushing bottled water on their darling sons and daughters.

The yellow bus stops directly in front of us. A few steps inside and Cathy and Nate are seated. Directly across from them, Sam and I plop ourselves down. The bus fills expeditiously. It circles back around Buffalo Soldier lot and proceeds to Ike Hall. As we approach, we see the line of people snakes around the bottom entrance, steps, and the front and right-side sidewalks.

We exit the bus and follow the sequence line of those before us. Standing at the end of the line, I'm already thinking that the morning is flying by. Where did yesterday go? Last week? Last month? We just celebrated Nate's high school graduation from the bleachers, watching the Somerset Area High School Golden Eagles' Class of 2017 graduation to being moments away from taking our seats in Eisenhower Hall.

Cadets in the red sash are guiding us along. Everyone is cordial. "Good morning, sir," "Hello, ma'am," they say politely.

A few steps up the next flight of stairs and we're greeted by an officer.

"Welcome! It's going to be an exciting day!" he says.

A smile ensues as he looks at Nate's long, full, curly head of hair.

"That's some nice hair," he jokingly adds on. He shakes Sam's hand and asks, "Do you have any plans to follow your brother to West Point?"

Sam shyly replies, "I'm thinking about it," all the while knowing it is not in his path. Sam has become used to this question, as everyone seems to ask it.

The doors open. It's refreshing to find ourselves in air-conditioning. It's going to be a tough day, and when all is said and done, it is most likely a blur. So this is R-Day!

Eisenhower Hall is inspiring, yet it carries an aura of intimidation as we look around the hall for the very first time. The Eisenhower Hall Theater is dedicated to bringing great performances to the United States Corps of Cadets, family, friends, and neighboring communities throughout the Hudson Valley and stretching to New York City and beyond. It's a showplace where Broadway plays, musicals, symphony orchestras, comedians, and country and rock stars perform. The stage has seen the likes of the Radio City Rockettes, Luciano Pavarotti, *Les Misérables*, Johnny Cash, Bob Hope, Dave Matthews Band, and *Hairspray*.

The theater is one of America's largest theater stages, second only to New York's Radio City Music Hall.

We're in! We walk down the aisle. We take our seats, approximately a third of the way in, facing stage right. The cadet candidates are being processed in groups of forty.

The theater doors close. Reality sets in. The line is moving too fast. Can we just freeze this moment in time? Please! It's as if all five senses are in play. Impressive sites of Ike Hall, the pictures on the walls, the enormity of the building itself. You hear everything yet nothing. We have a magnified focus on Nate. Cathy and I agreed beforehand that we would hold back our tears.

"Let's stay strong, upbeat, and positive, and give Nate a 'you got this' send-off!" she tells me. Good plan, and I completely agree.

There is a short briefing explaining the schedule of R-Day events and things to know. We know what is coming. We've seen the YouTube videos, and we've read about it. Now we are in the very midst of this moment.

It happens!

"You have sixty seconds to say goodbye," announces the briefing officer.

It is a tough moment for all. Mothers are crying. Lots of hugs. Handshakes. Pats on the back. Hands brushing across heads of hair. Cathy, Sam, and I each take our turn with our final hugs and kisses and goodbyes.

"We love you, Nate. You got this!"

"We'll be thinking about you and praying for you. Stay strong!"

Nate, not wanting to be at the end of the line, quickly exits the aisle to the right and makes his way to the front of the theater. He subtly glances back at us. We all smile. The door closes behind Nate and the other cadet candidates. It's 7:33 AM! Deep breaths and sighs. Now we begin to cry.

Nate is among more than 1,230 cadets selected from approximately 13,000 applicants. Nate's journey to West Point began one years ago when he made his first visit to the academy to attend West Point Summer Leaders Experience (SLE).

SLE is a highly competitive program where more than 6,000 applicants from across the United States compete for just 1,000 slots annually. SLE is targeted at high school juniors. The goal is to immerse these potential cadets into a one-week fast-paced experience consisting of academic classes, military training, physical fitness training, and intramural athletics. Nate was selected to attend SLE in June 2016. After he completed his week at West Point, he was sold.

"I want to go to West Point," he said. And one year later, July 3, 2017, is here. We are here. When we brought Nate to SLE, we stopped at the West Point Visitors Center to have our picture ID taken. Cathy told the person taking her picture that Nate was here for the week and hopeful that next year she would be back to have a parent ID taken for the Class of 2021.

Nate is off to begin the process of becoming a West Point cadet and future Army officer—administrative processing, initial issue and fitting of military clothing, the haircut, medical and physical evaluations, and marching, military courtesy, and discipline.

I think it's safe to say that discipline and yelling will be one in the same today.

Cathy calmly looks over the R-Day schedule. It is still early morning, close to 8:00 AM. Hungry, thirsty, tired, we're looking forward to some much-needed coffee. Luckily, the Association of West Point Graduates (AOG) is holding a different kind of reception.

We find our way to the outcrop of doughnuts, bagels, Danishes, blueberry and banana bread, fruit, water, orange juice, and, yes, coffee! Ike Hall is busy. The new cadet groupings are finding their way in and out of the theater hall.

As Cathy, Sam, and I sit with our juice and coffee, rehashing the events of the previous hour, we see red, teary-eyed moms, girlfriends, brothers, and sisters, etc., grabbing their coffee and juice. Very touching.

Upon finishing our Continental breakfast, we start to write what will be the first of many letters to Nate. This is all Cathy! This was all her idea. Well organized, planned out, and prepared, she brought three stamped envelopes and paper. She knew we would have time to fill the day. So being the perfect mom, she knew what we could do—sit, decompress a bit, and send Nate our thoughts of what we were going through on this R-Day. As it turned out, one of the display booths in Ike Hall was the US Postal Service.

There is a booth supported by cadets handing out address cards for the soon-to-be new cadets. Now we know how to address our envelopes! The company address and rooms are contained on a little address card. Now we get to mail our first letters! Perfect!

Also among the United States Postal Service was many West Point organizations from across the country, various vendors selling Class of 2021 and other USMA West Point clothing, and the Army A-Club.

The A-Club supports Army West Point Cadet-Athletes by generating financial support for the many Division I athletics sports teams.

And today, well, today is about bringing the newest members of the Army family into the fold. Translated, this means "Go Army, Beat Navy!" The two gentlemen manning the A-Club booth were all about the Army Black Knights repeating their 2016 football performance against Navy. A 21–17 win at M&T BANK stadium in Baltimore, Maryland, where Army ended a fourteen-year run of frustration against Navy. On December 10, 2016, and for the first time in fifteen years, Navy was the first to sing its alma mater after the game against Army.

That gloomy overcast distinction falls to the loser of one of college football's most storied rivalries. Sing second!

We shared our story about Nate to the A-Club gentleman about Somerset County and beautiful western Pennsylvania.

Now let's talk Army-Navy football tickets. We were easily sold on the Army A-Club membership.

Our first experience would come later that fall on October 21, 2017—a home game at Michie Stadium where the Black Knights went up against the Temple Owls. What a game! Army, trailing from behind, would complete a 79-yard scoring drive in the final 91 seconds and a final touchdown with one second left in regulation to tie the game at 28.

Army kicked a 29-yard field goal in the first overtime for a dramatic 31–28 victory on that amazing, sunny, autumn Saturday afternoon occurring on Family Weekend at West Point.

Here at Ike Hall, it's a seller's paradise! I pick up several items—a Class of 2021 T-shirt, West Point 1802 ball cap, a West Point license plate cover. Cathy and Sam make their hat selections. Great choices all around.

The sun is unimpeded today. Not a cloud in the sky. The hats will be must-haves later today. Still many hours until we find our way to the bleachers on the Plain to keep an eye out for Nate, our Plebe.

We continue to walk around various areas of Ike Hall. The line for parent-identification badges is incredibly long. I look at the schedule, and Cathy and I decide that we'll try closer to 2:00 PM when the ID center closes.

The chapel of the Most Holy Trinity at the United States Military Academy is a Catholic church and place of worship for many members of the Corps of Cadets. An 11:30 AM Mass is on the schedule for today followed by a luncheon hosted by Most Holy Trinity.

It's hard not to take in the beauty in history of the West Point grounds. Leaving Ike Hall, we slowly walk along Washington Road and circle back toward Trophy Point and the Overlook of the Hudson River and Constitution Island. We walk by the Thayer Monument, Battle Monument, and Sedgwick Monument. Like us, many people are simply walking the grounds, taking in the multitude of sites. We glance over and observe the Superintendent's Quarters and Commandant's Quarters. Your eyes are immediately drawn to the Beat Navy sign on the front of the Superintendent's Quarters. How cool!

We approach Holy Trinity Chapel and step inside. I know we are here to celebrate mass on this special day, but the first thing that runs through my mind is air-conditioning! It feels so good!

We take our seats in one of the pews halfway up in the church. And my second thought: it feels so good to sit down! My feet are aching from all the walking we've done so far today. Mass begins, celebrated by Most Holy Trinity's chaplain.

Father's homily touches upon everything we need to hear today. Turn our thoughts, concerns, our emotional roller coaster that we've been on, and faith into Jesus Christ's hands. His words have a calming tone, to the effect of your sons and daughters have chosen a path of service—as defenders of this country, side by side with their friends and fellow soldiers.

Soothing words at the right time. Like Cathy and me, I'm fairly certain that those seated with us in Holy Trinity Chapel are wondering what their cadet daughter or son is in the midst of at this moment.

Did my cadet get to eat lunch? How did the haircut go? Are you drinking water? Are you feeling okay? Is this what you really want to do? And even that out-in-left-field thought, are they being nice to you?

The chaplain, a colonel and West Point graduate himself, projects a much-needed message, "Everything will be all right." Many of us here at Mass today are in a new, uncharted territory, our first experiences with the ways of the military. And adding to those emotions is an extra heightened sense that our child is attending one of the most prestigious military academies in the world.

Written in history, world renowned, this is West Point, and our son is next to become a link in the Long Gray Line. Quite humbling. Proud doesn't even begin to convey and describe how we're feeling. It's a combination of both excitement and fear. Exciting because of Nate's decision to serve in the military and that element of fear because of what comes along with knowing that he will be put in harm's way. Gut-wrenching for any parent.

But this is why we're here at Mass. Catholic Mass is a celebration of the self-sacrifice of Jesus Christ. And today we stand in Holy Trinity Chapel at West Point to find ourselves as witness to His sacrifice. And as so often happens in our lives, we easily find the connection with being at Mass and knowing that Nate and the other cadets, on this special Reception Day, are committing themselves to a period of service by way of self-sacrifice to our nation.

Mass finishes. Up next, a luncheon hosted by a welcoming group from Holy Trinity. Cathy, Sam, and I make our way to the basement of the church. Everyone is cheerful and welcoming. The atmosphere is one of "the door is always open." Better yet, I'm thinking, *Hey, it's lunchtime.* Cheese, crackers, vegetables, dip, and a nice layout to make sandwiches. Ham, salami, turkey are part of the selection. I load up my plate, and we find a place to sit and eat.

"How are you holding up, Sam?" I ask.

"I'm good," Sam says.

Midday and we've been through a lot. I bring back a small plate of cookies for the three of us. The upside of having lunch at Holy Trinity and on West Point grounds is that we don't have to leave—no need to find a shuttle bus back to Buffalo Soldier Field parking lot or walk to someplace else within the USMA grounds.

So much walking. And in one of those uncanny, serendipitous moments, Sam speaks out, "I wonder how Little Buddy (our nickname for Cody) is doing!"

Cathy and I respond in similar fashion, "We were thinking the same thing."

We all smile.

The weather back home is nearly identical to what we are seeing here—high 80ºF, low 90ºF with high humidity. Hot, sticky, and sweaty. It's ironic to think that we have it tough, walking around, taking in the West Point sights and sounds, all the while we begin to see hints of what R-Day has in store for these new, incoming cadets.

We have it so rough. Uh-huh, sarcasm.

The echoes in the distance are evidence of what is taking place. The same sounds reverberate as we find ourselves between Thayer Hall and Cullum Hall. A short walk along the pathway toward the Eisenhower Monument past Jefferson Hall, a few pictures on our iPhones of the surrounding area and we come to the source of the sounds. Orderly yelling and screaming emanating from within canopies set up inside the Central Area, adjacent to Washington Hall. Cadets in the Red Sash, a.k.a. Firsties (First-Class Cadets), have found their rhythm. We look down the walkway by Nininger Hall and see some of the activity driving the racket.

Large green duffel bags being carried by cadets in T-shirts and black shorts. And perhaps one of the easiest and simplest one-line sentence to botch. How difficult can it be to remember a few words and recite them back when instructed? The new cadets can't move on till they report successfully, regardless of how many attempts are made. They are being prepped by other cadre.

"You will walk up to the Cadet in the Red Sash's line, stand at attention, render the proper salute. You will say 'Sir, new Cadet Doe reports to the Cadet in the Red Sash for the first time as ordered."

Another set of lines to wait in. Any waiting is just time for anxiety to rush in. The good news is, well, if there is good news for these young men and women is that the lines and processing are moving like well-oiled machines.

And then it comes. Those words. The shot heard round and round the central area. But a round is also a musical composition type. Wikipedia defines it as "a song which can be sung by two or more groups of people. One group starts off and the next group starts to sing the same song a bit later. It should sound nice together." This is where I end Wikipedia's description of a round. The *songs*, or words being sung by the Firsties, are anything but nice.

Phones are held high in the air, and pictures and recordings are set in motion. The sound echoes outward.

"New cadet! Step up to my line! Not on my line, not over my line, not behind my line! Step up to my line!" the experienced cadre yell.

We don't hear exactly what the cadet says. But the high-volume sounds of "What are your four responses?" are heard clearly.

Cathy, Sam, and I can hear various replies of "Yes, sir," "No, sir," "No excuse, sir," "Sir, I do not understand" among the many shaved, bald heads making their way through the lines.

We wonder, *Did Nate make it through on his first try?*

The sun is high in the sky, not a cloud to be seen. It is bright. The sun's rays are penetrating and beating down on my exposed neck and arms. My hat offers some relief, but my nose and cheeks begin to take on a cherry hue.

"How will all those newly shaved, glistening heads make out today?" Cathy, in a motherly fashion, says.

She hopes someone is keeping an eye on sunburns and providing sunscreen for the cadets. We can only hope.

We find some shade covering a few benches near Jefferson Hall and take a seat. A few drinks from our bottled waters and Cathy provides a reset on what is next.

"Let's walk back to Ike Hall," she says.

The photo ID badge line for the Class of 2021 cadet parents was meandering every which way earlier in the morning. The schedule says that the parent ID photos end at 2:00 PM. We take a twisting and serpentine path back to Ike Hall, slowly walking by Cullum and Lincoln halls toward Trophy Point.

Trophy Point gets its name from the numerous display pieces of captured artillery spanning back to the Revolutionary War. It is also the location of Battle Monument, one of the largest columns of granite in the world. It provides a breathtaking view of the Hudson River, and surrounding mountainsides oftentimes are seen as a potpourri of colors with the sunrise, sunset, and mix of cloud cover that varies with the seasons. A must-see!

Ten minutes before the ID center closes and we're in. And best of all, no line. What a difference from earlier this morning. Cathy and I complete the photograph identification form, and several minutes later, we each have in our possession Class of 2021 cadet parent identification cards, with an expiry date of 2021 June 1.

Sam has been a trooper through everything—all the walking, the early start, waiting in lines, talking to others like us; he's doing great. It's only been three months since his spinal fusion surgery.

"Sam, how are you feeling? Any pain?" Cathy asks.

"I'm good," he says.

I ask him if he wants to go back to the hotel room, and he simply says no. Any pain or discomfort he may be experiencing is being overshadowed by his separation from his best friend and brother. Not yet sixteen years old but he is our rock. Sam has a maturity beyond his fifteen and a half years.

"Are you up for barbecue later, Sam?" I ask. "We can try Barnstormers."

"Sure, that sounds good," he replies.

The upside is that Barnstormers is a short walk from the Holiday Inn Express where we are staying. We won't have to drive anywhere.

Up next on the schedule is the superintendent brief at 3:00 PM at the Eisenhower Hall. The fifty-ninth superintendent of the US Military Academy has a captive audience on this memorable July summer day. The auditorium is full. All eyes are fixed on the white screen projecting Welcome to the United States Military Academy Class of 2021.

The superintendent has been West Point superintendent since July 17, 2013. He himself is a 1975 West Point graduate, was commandant of cadets at the Academy from 2006 to 2008, and is an exemplary officer with a distinguished Army career.

His voice carries effortlessly through Eisenhower Theater's massive auditorium. His words are clear and crisp. His message radiates out words to the entire audience. He has our attention. It's only been a matter of hours since we said our goodbye to Nate, but we seem to be in information deprivation. We feel compelled to grab on to any and all tidbits, any factoids that we can link to our cadet.

I glanced around, and it seems like the entirety of this hall are all in familiar company. We are all part of a new extended family. Our common thread—our Class of 2021 cadet sons and daughters.

That sense of pride has almost materialized into some physical, tangible entity. It's such a good feeling!

The superintendent gives us a breakdown of the Class of 2021 by the numbers:

12,973 applicants
4,019 nominated
2,220 qualified
1,229 admitted
1247 SAT average
28 ACT average
86 valedictorians
147 class presidents
832 team captains
1,087 varsity letters
301 women (24.5%)
205 African Americans (16.7%)
120 Hispanics (9.8%)
100 Asians (8.1%)
13 international cadets
7 combat veterans

The incoming class eclipses highs for both women and African Americans. The superintendent's testament to this data results in a round of applause. The Class of 2021 includes cadets from every state in the nation and thirteen international cadets entering the class under the sponsorship of their respective countries.

The countries represented include Bangladesh, Bulgaria, Cameroon, Liberia, Malaysia, Moldova, Mongolia, Poland, Romania, South Korea, Taiwan, and Thailand. Upon graduation, these cadets will return to their respective countries as officers in their armed forces.

The superintendent continues speaking, providing a week-by-week overview of the cadet basic training (CBT) highlights that will occur over the following six weeks. CBT training is one of the most challenging events a cadet will encounter over the course of their four years at the academy.

The initial military training program provides cadets with basic skills to instill discipline, pride, cohesion, confidence, and a high sense of duty to prepare them for entry into the Corps of Cadets.

Areas of summer instruction over these upcoming July and August weeks will include first aid, mountaineering, hand grenades, rifle marksmanship, and nuclear, biological, and chemical training.

The completion of cadet basic training is culminated with a twelve-mile march from Camp Buckner on the west end of West Point to the military academy's central post. And most importantly, this is the lead into our first personal contact with Nate. The Saturday following March Back is Acceptance Day, A-Day, the first opportunity for the newly accepted cadets to see and spend time with their family and friends.

Go figure. We're not even finished getting through R-Day and the countdown to A-Day is underway. Separation is a tough thing. But a good thing as well. The separation of time and distance, texting, Snapchatting, Facebook posts will make that August reunion all the more special. We can hardly wait!

The superintendent seamlessly progresses through the remainder of the slide deck. Someone was in game-day mode because there are a lot of slides with pictures of today's cadet processing. Jumping on the bus, haircuts, pull-ups, clothing pickup.

"Hey," Sam belts out, "that's Nate! There, in the green shirt!"

"Holy cow, it is!" Cathy replies. "It is our Nate!"

Up on the auditorium screen is a slide of cadets seated on a bus, holding their personal belongings. No smiles. Eyes are looking forward, the look of what in the world is coming next?

It is such a cool feeling being able to see Nate. He's on his way—in the heart of R-Day processing and surviving. The mom in Cathy kicks in.

"I hope he's doing all right," she says.

The next slide only adds to her tension and perhaps one specific mom's concern.

The screen shows a picture of a female cadet with bloody knees. I think everyone's eyes are drawn to her knees.

"It looks like she may have fallen on the sidewalk or stairs," I say.

Easy enough to do, I imagine. All the cadets are carrying over-sized duffel bags and backpacks. Two hands and two arms aren't enough on a day like today.

Up next is the seventy-seventh commandant of the US Corps of Cadets who steps in and speaks to several of the slides. He goes into more detail for the cadet basic training program. Week one includes in-processing, equipment issue, diagnostic fitness test, swim test, academic placement testing, drill and ceremony, and physical fitness (PT).

Oh yes, PT! No shortage of PT during CBT. The commandant's words strike a similar tone to that of the superintendent. It is their honor to hold the responsibility of developing and mentoring the Army's future leaders and defenders of our great nation. Another flash of pride permeates the auditorium.

We all have smiles on the outside, but there is a sense of uncertainty still lingering, an element of finality still yet to come at day's end when we see the Class of 2021 march out onto the Plain.

The commandant's wife then steps up to the podium after the commandant gives her a touching, love-filled "she's my rock" introduction. Another round of applause fills the auditorium in Ike Hall. It's easy to see that they've been through a lot together, much more than what can be captured on a one-page biographical sheet.

They are no strangers to West Point. The commandant graduated from the US Military Academy in 1990 as an infantry officer, and his wife is also a USMA Class of 1990 graduate. And the Long Gray Line continues on with their son, who is currently attending the academy, another link in the Corps of Cadets.

So it's safe to say that they are in familiar and relatable territory standing before the observant and attentive Class of 2021 families.

The commandant's wife stands confidently before the podium in the auditorium in Ike Hall and just puts it out there: "I know how you feel." A few chuckles, a few nods of agreement. She goes on to reassure the audience that our sons and daughters are being well taken care of. It's been a busy day for sure, and the cadets won't remember much of what they actually went through, she indicates.

The superintendent's welcome finishes ahead of the scheduled 3:00 PM to 4:30 PM timeslot. It's 4:00 PM. Her final words tell us that she has firsthand experience that there will be plenty of seating for the oath ceremony on the Plain. The R-Day schedule list 6:30 PM for the oath ceremony. And she adds to please be seated by 6:00 PM.

I look at my watch, then lean into Cathy and Sam. "We have almost two hours. What should we do?" I ask.

Cathy says, "We should go find a seat on the bleachers. They're going to fill up fast."

No sooner than Cathy says this, the theater doors open and people are off to the races. Wow! Do they know something we don't? The crowd is exiting in a determined way. And we do the same. Better safe than sorry.

"Let's make our way up to the Plain," says Cathy. I agree.

Sam is all-in and quietly walks alongside of us. It's been a long and arduous day—physically and emotionally.

The Welcome Class of 2021 Reception Day schedule listed a jam-packed schedule of events. Tours of West Point, Constitution Island, self-tours of West Point cemetery and the West Point museum, and performances by the Hellcats West Point band at Trophy Point and Eisenhower Hall Theater. The Cadet chapel, Catholic chapel, and Jewish chapel, in addition to the many gift shops, were slotted on the things to do for R-Day. Where did the day go? How did we miss out on these?

We wind our way through Trophy Point and arrive at the bleachers overlooking the Plain. The mad dash from Ike Hall shows the seating in full swing. The bleachers are beginning to fill. The Plebe mailing-address card and company assignments provided earlier on the third level of Ike Hall is coming in handy now.

Nate is assigned to the E Company Second Platoon, or E-2. The bleacher sections are lettered into groups, A–D and E–I. Fantastic! The oath ceremony legend on the back of the Reception Day schedule pamphlet makes sense now.

Everyone is in "locate your cadet" mode! The bleacher section is adjacent to the superintendent's review box. Cathy, Sam, and I find seats about two-thirds of the way up on the bleachers and take our seats. The countdown begins.

As it would be, the bleachers are facing in a southwesterly direction. The mid-to-late-day afternoon sun and its penetrating rays are indiscriminating. Sunscreen of all varieties is being applied. Sunglasses, umbrellas, ball caps, and bottled water are widespread.

Luckily, Cathy brought her wide-brimmed white beach hat, primarily so Nate could find us and, secondly, to provide coverage for her nose, cheeks, forehead, and neck. Looking around us, we're already seeing sunburn taking its toll.

Bottled water and snow cones are in high demand. There are several concession trailers set up behind the bleachers and I make my way back to pick up a few things. I wait my turn in line and place my order.

"Two bottled waters, two snow cones, and two soft pretzels please," I politely ask.

I take my order and walk a few steps and flop. I drop one of the soft pretzels. Darn! I quickly make my way back to Cathy and Sam and share my *drop* story. They take it all in stride. Smiles on their faces. Neither of them wanted a pretzel, so the lone survivor is mine. They happily take the snow cones from me. And between the bottled water and snow cones, we find some relief from the unrelenting sun and heat.

Here we are. Seated in the bleachers on the Plain, the parade field at the United States Military Academy at West Point. It is an amazing site!

The flat terrain of the Plain stands out in contrast to the varied and hilly terrain of the surrounding academy grounds. A beautiful place! Incredible structures, buildings, sceneries encircled with majestic buildings full of history and legends. In a matter of minutes, our son, Nate, will be among an elite group on the parade grounds.

It begins.

The culmination of R-Day is here! This group of cadet candidates are nearing the end of their first day in the process of becoming West Point cadets and future US Army officers. We are bursting with pride for Nate!

The cadets are grouped by company and platoon in alphabetical company order and lead by guidon bearers. The order is A1 (A Company, First Platoon), A2, A3, A4, B1, B2, and so on to I4. The platoons are arranged by height, from the tallest in the front right to shortest in the rear left.

The band begins to play, and the parade announcements are being blasted through the speaker system. Then it happens!

We begin to catch glimpses of the gathering of uniformed young men and women at the sally ports. The companies and platoons grow in number, and they move in cadence to the crisp march of formation as they pass the review stand and find their place on the Plain. I struggle not to be overcome as the E Company Second Platoon marches in front of us to no avail. Both Cathy and I have tears in our eyes. Sam is video recording and also taking photographs. We scan the E-2 formation on the Plain repeatedly.

Then finally!

"I think I see Nate!" I tell Cathy and Sam. "Four rows back, fifth person in," I say.

I'm pretty certain it is him. But there are so many clean-shaved heads. I stick to my positive vibes and hold firm that, yes, I saw Nate. How thrilling!

I chuckle and share my inside joke with Cathy and Sam. I tell them I don't think I've ever heard so many references to Where's Waldo? before. The entire crowd of family and friends seated in the bleachers and along the walkways are caught up in the same game—where is my cadet?

Both Cathy and Sam are adept camera virtuosos. Cathy comments that she has over three hundred photographs to look over when we get back home. Then we'll need to scan through Sam's pics as well and whatever other photos that get shared on the social media pages and elsewhere. The entire class of 2021 extended family now shares a common bond. First order of business, find my cadet!

The superintendent sent each candidate for the Class of 2021 a letter with the Honor Code and the Cadet Creed, expectations all cadets must live by. He instructed them to memorize them before R-Day. Another letter arrived which cited the Army regulations and physical demands, explaining what they are. If the candidates could not perform such physical requirements on R-Day, they could be dismissed.

Cadet Honor Code

A cadet will not lie, cheat, steal, or tolerate those who do.

Cadet Creed

As a future officer,
I am committed to the values of Duty, Honor, Country.
I am an inspiring member of the Army profession, dedicated to serve and earn the trust of the American people.
It is my duty to maintain the honor of the Corps.
I will live above the common level of life, and have the courage to choose the harder right over the easier wrong.
I will live with honor and integrity, scorn injustice, and always confront substandard behavior.
I will persevere through adversity and recover from failure.
I will embrace the Warrior Ethos, and pursue excellence in everything I do.
I am a future officer and member of the Long Gray Line.

Duty • Honor • Country

And after a long, agenda-packed, and emotional day, the moment is here.

The commandant of cadets of the United States Military Academy at West Point leads the Oath of Allegiance. He firmly announces that "until now your son or daughter has been called cadet candidate. After they take the oath, they will be a new cadet."

Everyone in attendance arises. And cadets' hands are raised as they join in the oath.

"I (state your name), do solemnly swear that I will support the Constitution of the United States, and bear true allegiance to the national government; that I will maintain and defend the sovereignty of the United States, paramount to any and all allegiance, sovereignty, or fealty I may owe to any state or country whatsoever; and that I will at all times obey the legal orders of my superior officers, and the Uniform Code of Military Justice."

The new cadets, having been received into their summer training companies, newly shorn and uniformly clad, now march off the Plain in a long gray line and through the double doors of Washington Hall.

We are awestruck and held spellbound by the view of the Corps of Cadets marching away. The history and the significance of this moment leave us humbled, honored, and proud.

Nate has joined the venerated institution that is West Point, ground that has been walked by US presidents, astronauts, heads of state, Medal of Honor recipients, Rhodes scholars, and Heisman Trophy winners. He is embarking on a journey traveled by some of our nation's most esteemed leaders.

But this R-Day would not end without fanfare. As the Corps of Cadets march in single file toward the tall wooden doors of Washington Hall, it happens!

The sprinkler system begins to spray streams of water in front of the bleachers and the review stand! Directly spraying and soaking the six executive officers, including the superintendent, commandant, dean of the academic board, and the command sergeant major.

No one is spared! But to the surprise and amazement of the crowd, not one of them flinches or moves, standing tall and firm, eyes straightforward, as they continue to watch like statues as the last of the Corps of Cadets passed through the doors of Washington Hall.

Talk about discipline! It's as if the shadowed images of these cadets are slowly evaporating. Now they are all gone. The Plain is empty. No band, no marching, no cadence, and no Nate in sight.

Thump! The doors to Washington Hall close.

And so, ends Reception Day, R-Day, for Nate and the West Point Class of 2021.

When will we next hear from Nate?

The waiting begins.

CHAPTER 3

We've Got Mail

"CAN I START you off with something to drink?" the waitress at Barnstormer's Barbeque asks.

"A margarita please and ice water for all of us," Cathy says.

"I'll try the Allagash," I thirstily reply. It's a white Belgian wheat beer. "And the coldest one you've got!"

Sam is the last to order. "Mountain Dew please," he asks politely.

We sit back, and in sync, we all take a deep breath and breathe a sigh of relief. Surviving R-Day as family members had its emotional ups and downs—final goodbyes, lots of walking, the element of the unknown of a Class of 2021 cadet. It is now 8:39 PM, Monday, July 3, 2017, and Cathy and I take a drink from our frosted glasses. We say a prayer of thanks and make a toast to the new cadets. "Cheers!" We look around at those seated in the less-than-spacious dining area, smelling of delicious BBQ sauces and smoky flavors, and see the looks of faces matching how we feel.

"How's your back?" Cathy leans in to Sam, motherly checking in on him. It's been a long two days, little rest and an emotional roller-coaster ride for everyone.

Just a few days over three months since Sam's spinal fusion surgery. He's been a real trooper today.

49

Now a quick check of the menu, a delectable selection of barbe-cue chicken, sandwiches, ribs, brisket, and barbecue combos.

Sam zeroes in on the BBQ pulled pork sandwich and french fries. Cathy and I look over the pick-your-own-barbecue combos, and we each select two meats. Cathy goes with the pulled pork and brisket, and I choose the kielbasa and brisket.

The dining area and the nearby surroundings from the Holiday Inn Express to Barnstormer's carries a savory, spicy, sweet, enticing, and tempting aroma.

Here comes the corn bread! "Oh my goodness!" I tell Cathy and Sam. "This corn bread is delicious."

I continue to rave about how tasty the cornbread is to the point where Cathy says, "Let's just order some for you later."

* * *

We've only made one return visit to Barnstormer's BBQ since that R-Day visit. It was a late April 2018 gathering with Nate and several of his cadet friends from E-2. We made the trip to West Point to watch Nate and his fellow club soccer teammates take on Navy on that clear but cool and crisp Saturday afternoon. The Black Knights came up short in a 2–1 loss to Navy on that day. Oh well.

Nate and his buddies were thrilled to be bypassing whatever Washington Hall had in store for them. They looked ravenous and microscopically eyed the menu. I swear they were all drooling.

And at that moment, both Cathy and Sam took the opportu-nity to take their potshots at me and share my corn bread infatuation with the cadets, reminiscing back to that R-day dinner.

Dining adjacent to us on that April 2018 evening were three other Plebe cadets. They were nearing the end of their meals when our waitress checked on us. I quietly leaned and asked her to add their dining bill to mine and not to let them know.

Before too long, these three cadets finished and began looking around, surprised to find that their meals were taken care of, their tab paid. The dining room was packed that evening, conversations loud, and plenty of drinks being indulged upon. Yet these three sharply dressed Plebes, looking strong and proud, somehow knew that it was me.

They stood up, pushed their chairs into the table, took a few steps toward Cathy and me, and, with wide-brimmed smiles, politely acknowledged us and said, "Thank you. That was very kind of you."

It's my hope that this evening experience made its way back to their parents, family, and others, letting the many loved ones know that the West Point family of families extended a small gesture of simple kindness. It warms the heart and soul.

* * *

"What do you think Nate is doing now?" asks Cathy.

"I'm not sure," I reply. "But after such a busy day, I can't imagine them going too much longer with any kind of additional R-Day stuff."

"I'm full," Sam calls out.

"That was really, really good," I say.

And Cathy makes it unanimous. "Yes, it was." With that said, we depart Barnstormer's, and our penultimate R-Day activity comes to an end. Exhausted, we make the short walk back to the hotel.

Reception Day, July 3, 2017, at West Point is finished—for us anyway. For the Class of 2021, up next is six weeks of Beast Barracks.

"Good morning, Sam," Cathy greets Sam. "Happy Fourth of July!"

"Happy Fourth, Mom," Sam replies in a still overly tired manner.

"We'll probably pass some fireworks vendors along the way, and we can pick up a few things to set off later tonight," I tell Sam.

Hillary was the first to leave the nest. Nate has the next forty-seven months mapped out, and that leaves Sam. He is our focus now.

New beginnings and the ever-changing dynamics of what life's pathways have in store for our family. It's like a countdown to a rocket launch—5, 4, 3, 2, 1!

Five. For the longest time it was the five of us, dragging Nate and Sam along to sit in the bleachers and watch Hillary play basketball, tennis, and softball. Not too long ago, it was her graduation from the University of Pittsburgh at Johnstown, Pennsylvania, ceremony. And last November, a beautiful sun-filled, blue-sky day—her wedding day.

Up next, in a few days, we'll be moving her and Jacob into their first house, a quaint, well-kept three-bedroom colonial home in Chambersburg, Pennsylvania. Moving day is Saturday, July 8, 2017.

Nate was apologetic to Hillary prior to leaving for R-Day. Sorry that he wouldn't be there to help with the move. Hillary reassured him that all would be okay.

"Nate, you got this! You can visit when you get your first break," she lovingly told him.

The love between a brother and sister—genuine, caring, and selfless.

And perhaps in selfish retrospect, I think, *We did something right.* Just look at these kids. Hillary, in her typical, loving fashion and maturity often tells us, "you don't spoil us, you just eliminate all the obstacles to help us succeed." I can't help but smile.

Four. The boys have always outnumbered the girls, 3–2. But now, Cathy stands in at a 3–1 disadvantage. Boys rule! Sam, Nate, and I have done our best to keep Mom the center of attention; she's the foundation of our family.

Cathy and I are a way off from being tagged as empty nesters. Two high school boys make for no shortage of excitement. West Penn Soccer games, traveling to various places in the Pittsburgh vicinity, along with Sam and Nate both being certified as US Soccer Federation referees for Western Pennsylvania, weekends were always booked.

Soccer games covering both spring and fall, and throw in football, hockey, and tennis to finish out the boys' sports involvement. Oh, we can't forget guitar lessons in the mix too. I always enjoyed listening to the boys play.

But from this R-Day perspective, those activities and thoughts and memories seem like a lifetime ago. Nate has moved on the next chapter in his journey. And now...

Three. Yes, it is now the three of us. In some ways, I think Sam is dreading being caught in the middle of us, that is, Mom and Dad. But at the same time, I think Sam will welcome the attention. It's too easy to forget that we're all in the midst of separation anxiety. Nate and Sam had each other to lean on when Hillary left for college and then when she got married. Now Sam is going at it alone. One sister and one brother moving on in the next steps in their lives, as is Sam. He's all Mom and Dad's now.

On this July 4 return trip back to Friedens, Pennsylvania, we decide to forgo our typical route cutting across I-81 to I-80 and south past State College. Today, our plan is to take I-81 toward Harrisburg and catch the Pennsylvania turnpike, I-76.

"Let's mix it up a little," I say. "We can stop at Taco Bell, Sam. And we'll probably find someone selling fireworks."

Cathy is rather pensive. Understandably so. R-Day was a trying event, and the buildup and culmination of our final goodbye to Nate has now provided an opening to that pressure relief valve. We can let our guards down! Whew!

In typical fashion, Sam is out cold. Once we start driving, his headset goes on, head tilted back, and eyes close.

How many times have we seen this before? Plenty. The only difference on this trip is that familiar brotherly face is not next to him. He and Nate are mirror images of each other when they're in the back seat.

The miles go quickly by, and before I know it, Taco Bell time. Honestly, I don't know what Sam, and for that matter, Nate, too, see in the Taco Bell cuisine. Don't get me wrong. I'm not trying to bash Taco Bell; perhaps it's a dining pleasure better suited to the younger crowd.

"Here we are, Sam. Time to grab a bite to eat," I tell him. I see the look in Cathy's eyes and can tell she's just as excited as I am for one of the combination meals. Yet here we are, and we make the most of it. And better still, as I predicted, fireworks—directly across from the Taco Bell parking lot.

Two. Soon, Sam will be heading to college and Cathy and I will be empty nesters.

One. Our attention will turn to the only one left at home—Cody. Daily walks and playful exchanges with our lil' buddy.

And our lunch conversation turns to Cody.

"We'll save some of the bottle rockets and Roman candles for Cody," Sam deviously says.

Sam is up to no good. How can he even imagine such a thing? I think he wants to see how riled and excited Cody reacts to the fireworks.

Why not? I think to myself. It'll have to wait until tomorrow when we pick Cody up from May's Country Kennels. We peruse the tent, eyeing what is discounted and purchase two combo packs. Sam is pleased. The thought of lighting fireworks in the backyard tonight brings some sense of normalcy to the day. Things are different. I know it, Cathy knows it. And Sam is showing it. We are three.

Making the turn into our driveway is surreal; the last three days are fresh in our minds, but a lot of what we went through is still a blur. I'm sure there is some medical or psychological term for what we're feeling. But I simply chalk it up to two things: we are tired, and we miss our Nate. No words ring truer as we open the car doors and begin to unpack the car. "There's no place like home."

And like Dorothy from *The Wizard of Oz*, we click our imaginary ruby slippers. There's definitely something to be said about familiarity. It sure does feel good to be back home, laundry being the exception. The air-conditioning is running and provides a comforting blanket of coolness. These last two days have taken a toll on us emotionally, without a doubt. And physically too. It'll be interesting to check our step count. Admittedly, it feels good to kick back in our home surroundings. Home sweet home—cool, comforting, relaxing, and all the amenities that come with our sweet abode. That is, less one person.

Cathy is the first to say it. "I wonder what Nate is doing now."

It's after 6:00 PM this July 4 evening. We order from Pizza Hut to keep dinner simple. No cooking and cleanup is a few paper plates and napkins tossed into the garbage. Easy enough.

Sunset and complete darkness are quickly fading and take us into a countdown. T minus two hours.

Go figure. Three hours later and no fireworks. They will have to wait. We're too tired and the air-conditioning feels too good. Tomorrow. We convince ourselves that one more day won't matter. Who cares? Plus, Cody isn't here either.

July 4, 2017, comes and goes without much fanfare. Saturday, July 8, is the next big day for us. Moving day.

Hillary and Jacob have taken the next big step in their young lives—homeowners. Cathy, Sam, Pap, and I, along with Jacob's mom and dad, have been officially recruited as movers. No problem. We've been there plenty of times before. Hillary is so excited, moving from their apartment to a house with a yard. Stella and Remi will have some freedom. Wednesday, Thursday, and Friday fly by. Once again, we find ourselves in the car, traveling down the turnpike. And once again, moving day, as so many other days, turns into a thing of the past. It was a hot and humid day. A lot of sweating for sure. I can't even begin to imagine how many trips I made up and down the stairs. How many boxes did we carry? How many trips to the U-Haul? How many this? How many of that? It doesn't matter now. The good news and most important takeaway is that Hillary and Jacob are certified homeowners—mortgage, yard, garden, lawnmower, and all. Wonderful and exciting times, even freshly cut grass clippings.

All in all, it wasn't a bad day. We make our way back to Somerset, Pennsylvania, by early evening.

"Pap, would you like to eat dinner at Rey Azteca?" Cathy inquires.

Sam's eyes open, and his ears easily pick up Cathy's invitation to Pap. Cathy quaintly convinces Pap to join us for dinner; local Mexican cuisine is the overwhelming choice after finishing our moving-day commitment for Hillary and Jacob.

The four of us are absorbed into our seats. Body aches, sore muscles, stiff arms and legs, and tightened muscles in our backs are overtaking us. Eating out was a good choice! And our conversation turns to the events of day, smiles and joy for the new homeowners.

Being busy has been the order of the day. Go, go, go. At least that's how it seemed. But the time certainly flew by in all the excitement—physically draining tied with emotional highs!

Now, yes, now. What about Nate? What is he doing at this very moment? What's in store? His first weekend at West Point. What do they do with 1,200-plus new faces on a Saturday evening?

Luckily for us, the answer is uncomplicatedly being streamed live on Facebook.

Cathy and I lackadaisically, or perhaps, in more of an overtaxed manner, find our way to the common Olsavsky gathering place: the kitchen table.

The laptop comes out and is powered up. YouTube, Facebook, the West Point Moms' page, and many other online sources have been our go-to places for any tidbits regarding our Plebe. What a whirlwind these last few days have turned out to be.

It's interesting and, to some extent, fascinating to reflect on the events of that first week of July 2017. Three topics immediately come to mind. First, Nate and West Point. Second, moving day for Hillary and Jacob, where they now call Chambersburg, Pennsylvania, home. And third, the weather. Yes, of all things, the weather. Here I am, two years later, still thinking of that stifling hot, humid July summertime mix of Mother Nature's elements.

Saturday, July 8, 2017, showed a high of 86°F with a low temperature of 71°F with a relative humidity of 65°. How do I know this, you ask? Well, I have an instant recall memory! Uh, not quite. To be honest, I searched the daily weather archives from the Pennsylvania State Climatologist website at climate.psu.edu. Chuckle, chuckle.

But this Saturday evening is different. No break, the air is calm. The black-and-gold West Point flag, along with the US flag, droop from the left side of the front porch. The colors are clearer, crisper—red, like crimson; white, the immaculate; and the blue, like deep crystalline sapphire! The stars and stripes have aggrandized our sense of pride more so than ever before. Our Plebe has brought this new-found heightened awareness to us. What a great feeling! Duty, honor, country. Those three words now resonate passionately within us.

The game of find my cadet is in full swing once again. Cathy is live streaming the Fourth of July celebration at Trophy Point. Nate and his fellow Class of 2021 cadets are marching to the cheers and applause of family, friends, and others from the Highland Falls and surrounding communities. Each company being led by Firsties, fourth-year cadets, and Cows, third-year cadets.

Canteens are hanging from each cadet's left side. I'm pretty sure "stay hydrated" has been the orders of the day. Heads are shaved, and many are bearing the effects of too much sun. The procession continues on for over twenty-five minutes. The West Point Hellcats, the academy's field music group, play on and on and on. The drums and the drumsticks continue until each and every cadet finds his way to chairs specifically placed out for them.

The superintendent and commandant greet the Class of 2021 and the many hundreds and hundreds of onlookers in attendance.

"Welcome," the Superintendent succinctly says. "And at ease," he goes on to say. "This is your evening and you can officially stand down. Relax, breathe easy, and enjoy the evening." His words are well received. We see legs stretched out, arms being crossed, shoulders dropping, and smiles spreading across the cadet multitude.

Like us, I believe other cadet parents are finding some semblance of comfort and consolation in seeing that our cadets are relaxing, if only for an evening.

We watch early evening turn into sunset and then into nightfall. The Benny Havens Band, the popular music ensemble primarily serving the United States Corps of Cadets at West Point, are front and center onstage at Trophy Point. The cadets and everyone else on the hillside are enjoying the band's electrified best of rock, hip-hop, R & B, and country songs. Looks like a fantastic night!

R-Day plus a week. Finally, it happens. The US Postal Service delivers a much-anticipated stationery-size envelope:

From: Cadet Nathaniel Olsavsky, PO Box 3502, West Point, NY 10997-3502
To: Olsavsky Family

We've got mail! Our first letter from Nate! The excitement is beyond words. We've played the lottery from time to time over the years when the jackpot would top some mega-million-dollar number. Getting that first letter was on par with hitting the lottery. But unlike having Nate's letter in our hands, we've never hit the lotto. Regardless, the moment is priceless!

We've shared Nate's West Point address with family and friends. And to save him from any grief or embarrassment, we repeat the same instructions—plain white envelope, nothing colorful or glaring, make it to the attention of New Cadet Nathaniel Olsavsky. There are so many people sharing in our excitement, and our separation, who want to send words of encouragement to Nate. Very warming.

Letters have been going out on a continuing basis since returning home. Cathy has been on an almost-daily letter-writing pace. My tempo has been more in line with every two to three days.

It's been countless years since I last put pen to paper to write a letter. Cell phones, text messages, and social media have, to a great extent, depersonalized how we communicate. But now, yes, now we're back to writing letters, an age-old pastime of not so long ago. Admittedly, it takes some discipline to dedicate quiet time to gather your thoughts and craft them into words and sentences and stories, deciding on what color pen you'll use, plain stationery or something colorful, and actually addressing an envelope and putting a postage stamp on it.

R-Day and Beast have revived the lost art of letter writing for us. There is something inherently special and intimate about receiving a real handwritten letter. Time and distance are bridged knowing that someone took time to sit down to write a letter, fold it over, place a stamp on the envelope, and place it in their mailbox or drop it off at the nearest post office.

We're doing our best to keep Nate up-to-date on the latest events at home and in nearby Somerset. Sometimes our letters read like a restaurant's menu: crab legs, corn on the cob, watermelon, and peach cobbler. What is Nate having for dinner? Does he have time to eat? Is he losing weight? How is his spirit and morale? So many questions running through our minds.

The cadet basic training highlights presentation from the superintendent's brief is a constant go-to source of information—a week-by-week, play-by-play timeline of what the cadets are doing: swim test, drill and ceremony, basic rifle marksmanship, marching, land navigation, live fire, House of Tears, and more. Wow! A lot to take in. Times have changed. We're still in the midst of grasping that our son is in the Army. And not just the Army, he's attending one of the most elite institutions in the world—West Point!

Letters are going out; even Sam is writing. It's so cool to see him writing, something other than a school assignment, something different than a text or Snapchat. I believe this simple act of jotting a few words down on paper to his brother is comforting in its own way for him as well. To give and to receive.

It's easy to connect our faith, our connection to St. Peter's parish in Somerset, and Sam and Nate's time at St. Peter's School.

In every way, I have shown you that by hard work of that sort we must help the weak, and keep in mind the words of the Lord Jesus who himself said, "It is more blessed to give than to receive" (Acts of the Apostles 20:35)!

Sure, they're only letters. But still, they represent a connection of family, love, warmth, pride, and accomplishment.

Make no mistake, we are all being bolstered and encouraged by our newfound craft: pen, paper, envelopes, and stamps.

The traffic flow is definitely one-sided. Understandably so. We're just hoping for a few morsels of information from Nate. Anything will do. Even the extended Class of 2021 families are aligned. Many are facing empty mailboxes. No postcard, no letter, no word from our children. A relatable event. We're all experiencing the same emotions.

The next update from our cadet brings smiles to our faces. A brief note dated July 18, 2017: *Hi, family, I qualified earlier today. You need to hit 22/40 targets and it took me two tries. The first time I shot, I got 19/40; my second time I got 26/40. I AM PUMPED!*

Nate goes on to tell us that he felt like this was his first big accomplishment at West Point. Also, he was told that he passed the PT test the first week of CBT too. Lastly, Nate includes a postscript: *PS: A kid just rapped happy birthday to a girl and it was* crazy!

Our anxiety, jitters, doubt, and apprehension are put at ease with a short, crisp note. Our smiles are back, chins up, and we feel less angst.

New Cadet Olsavsky is doing just fine. But questions still abound. What is next? How is CBT going? Any injuries? Is training everything you thought it would be?

Any conversation of length covering details and everything else will have to wait until A-Day.

Waiting seems to be the operative word. A lot of things have come and gone.

- SLE
- Soccer camp at West Point
- Opening the candidate questionnaire
- Nomination applications
- Congressional interviews
- Nomination
- Official appointment letter
- High school graduation
- R-Day

What's a little more waiting?

Cadet basic training is all spelled out. The structure, the activities, the who, what, where, and when are all defined, which is a good thing, particularly as we approach the next key milestone—the two-minute check-in call.

As we understand it, the new cadets will be able to reach out for a very brief phone call. They'll most likely use their platoon leader's phone. So we're told to be on the lookout for an incoming call during week two of CBT.

I don't think we've ever been more connected to our cell phones; the anticipation is crushing. It comes on the evening of July 11, 2017. Finally!

Nate: Hi! How's it going?
Cathy: Hi, Nate! It's so good to hear from you.
Sam: Hi, Nate!
Cathy: We love you and miss so much.
Nate: I love you guys too! I have two minutes.

Cathy: Great, tell me all about everything. Do you need anything?

Nate: No, um, I'll send you guys a letter. Let me know if you guys are getting my letters.

Cathy and Joe: Oh yeah, we're getting them. One today and one yesterday.

Nate: Okay, good. I sent a bunch out today and yesterday, so you should be getting some more. And I'm going to write some more tonight too.

Cathy: You sound so good.

Nate: You guys sound good, too, just different. And I miss you, guys.

Cathy: Awe, miss you.

Nate: Hi, Sam! Hi, Dad! Tell everyone I said hi, all the friends and relatives and whoever is asking.

Joe: Cody just grabbed a napkin out of the garbage can. (*Laughter for everyone.*)

Cathy: So tell us about it!

Nate: Um, I don't know. Just been sitting in lines a lot. Got all our uniforms. Oh, oh, send me a letter with what we're doing for each of the six weeks. I want to know what we'll be doing.

Cathy, Joe: Okay.

Nate: You sent me the two weeks and that was great. I'd say PT is the worst part. Our waking up in the morning because we just get yelled at a ton. And then we did our three-mile march, so that was good. But we have to pack our stuff for that, and I just got done doing that. And it's just really hot here too and we're constantly sweating. They yell at us a lot, but the punishment isn't too bad. They're just mad a lot. (*Laughter and chuckles.*)

Joe: That's all part of it. And how are your feet? Okay?

Nate: Yeah, okay, no injuries. I'm just tired.

Joe: Are your shoes okay?

Nate: Yeah. We're authorized one piece of fruit in our room, and that's all we can have, no sweets. Some people got caught yesterday, and we got in trouble. (*More laughing.*) I'm writing you guys letters, and I'll keep you updated. I'm writing in my journal too.

Cathy: Are you getting our letters?

Nate: Yeah. They're great. Keep them coming. And they're really nice. They cheer me up.

Cathy: Okay, good. We're praying for you and thinking about you, sweetheart. Nothing going on back home. You're not missing much.

Nate: All right. I love you, guys. I gotta go. Keep the letters up, and I'll write to you, guys. We get a half-hour phone call soon.

Cathy: You're doing great! Keep up the good work.

Nate: I'll be calling in about two weeks.

Cathy: Yeah, the ice-cream social.

Nate: Yeah, that's it. I love you, guys.

Cathy, Joe, and Sam: Love you, Nate.

Joe: We're so proud of you!

Nate: Thanks. All right.

Joe: Okay, be safe.

Nate: Okay, I will be.

Everyone: Love you, bye.

Cathy checks out her library of pictures. And then she finds a few pics of Cody sitting on a chair, looking out the dining room window, standing at attention. She smiles and simply says, "Check out Cadet Cody."

The name sticks!

Our family canine is fully immersed in the West Point saga.

And then someone blurts out, not sure if it was Sam or Cathy or me, "Let's keep Nate up-to-date with the adventures of Cadet Cody. Send Nate some pictures, include some colorful dialogue, and make a few jokes about Cody's daily antics. Yes, this will work."

Cadet Cody is born! The adventures of Cadet Cody comes to life! The very first volume, surprisingly, comes into form without a hitch.

Five pictures: Cody at the window, three of me walking through the front door with mail, and a picture of Stella and Remi at their new homestead in Chambersburg, Pennsylvania. I cut and paste the pics into a Word document and insert callout balloons to add text;

amusing ad lib quips hem in the scenes. Volume 1 of *The Adventures of Cadet Cody* is christened on July 24, 2017. A story is born.

Roll the credits, I laughingly think out load. Not really. But now we have a fun, creative, different way to send Nate updates and news from the home front. It's a good feeling when we finish a letter to send to our cadet. Hard to describe, but it almost seems like a warm blanket being wrapped around your shoulders, if but for a moment, when the letter is placed in the mailbox, knowing that it will be received with comfort, satisfaction, and amusement.

The notes from Nate continue to trickle in. Of course, not to our satisfaction. That is, we would like more. More, more, more. More letters, more details, just more of what Nate is experiencing.

And Nate delivers with the ghostly and spectral tale about New Cadet Stanley.

"I have another story to tell you too!" Nate writes.

And Sam: "You better be reading this, too, Mister! I miss you!" he says.

Nate begins by describing how the cadets line up in the hallways—gear on, camelbacks, and heels flush against the wall. "This kills your calves, and after a few minutes, it makes them really sore and you start to cramp," Nate graphically describes the scene to us. "The first sergeant was yelling at all of us today. He caught me with my heels not on the wall."

Uh-oh, I think.

Nate tells us his punishment was to write a one-page paper. The topic: Cadet Stanley.

Nate writes, "First sergeant told us that Stanley was a new cadet a long time ago. Like me, Stanley didn't have his heels on the wall and his first sergeant caught him. Instantly, as Stanley stared into first sergeant's burning eyes, he was vaporized. All that remained of Stanley were his dog tags, which were given to his mother. And Stanley's soul was sucked straight into the Corps of Cadets!"

Nate has our attention and our smiles and grins with this letter. Interesting? Yes!

He goes on, "It's said that Stanley haunts the walls and inflicts his wrath on other new cadets by giving them pain in their calves."

We smile and chuckle. There's a *cuteness* to his words, but we know there is seriousness in the undertones of the messaging and training.

"But yeah, that's what I had to write. We get yelled at a lot, but the punishments aren't bad at all!"

Pretty cool stuff. We can't complain. Here we are, doing our best to send words of encouragement and all the latest happenings from home in the hope of winning a few smiles from our cadet. And what does he do?

Nate provides us with the reciprocal faultless dispatch of words that we intended to deliver. He comforts us, he brings smiles to our faces, and he warms our hearts. Crazy how things work out sometimes. Crazy in a good, super-rewarding way.

Up next, the ice-cream social. Midway through Beast Barracks, CBT is at the three-week point. And most importantly, we get to hear from Nate.

This is a special day for new cadets. They get the opportunity to go to the homes of sponsors in Highland Falls and nearby communities—TAC officers, West Point instructors and coaches—to enjoy the annual ice-cream social, technically called Quarters Visitation Day.

Basically, the ice-cream social gets new cadets out of CBT for a few hours to eat, drink refreshments, meet other new cadets, and make the much-anticipated phone calls home. It also gives the academy time for the change of cadre.

Yes, a live phone call! A chance to speak with Nate. We can't wait.

The day is Sunday, July 23, 2017, almost three weeks since we said our goodbyes. The Class of 2021 calendar, along with Nate sharing how this will go down, marks the moment. The time where the new cadets get but a brief respite from CBT challenges.

The West Point Moms' page is full of frenzied and elated exchanges simply because today is when we once again hear the voices of our beloved and much missed sons and daughters. No longer young boys and girls. No longer high school graduates. Now we are connecting to those brave few who are next in line—the Long Gray Line.

The instructions are straightforward: keep your phone close by. The call can come anytime, near noon (EST). And the phone number most likely won't be from someone we recognize.

A little after 1:00 PM, it happens!

"Hi, Mom," Nate says.

"Nate, how are you?" Cathy quickly rattles off. "It's so nice to hear you! We miss you. How are things going?"

"I'm with four other cadets," Nate explains. "We're at our sponsor's house, an officer. He's a major. They have three kids, two toddlers, and a little baby!" Nate tells us. "I'm calling from the baby's room."

"I can talk for a while, but we're all sharing the phone. I can FaceTime you guys, though, in a bit!" he says. "We're having a cookout. It's so good! I had two hamburgers, a Coke, and two brownies, and they have hot dogs, too, that I'll try."

Nate tells us that he and the other cadets are taking turns making phone calls and that he'll be able to FaceTime a bit later. *How cool!* we think.

We keep telling ourselves we are halfway through Beast. The good news, of course, is that Nate sounds great and seems to be in good spirits.

Honestly, the most difficult part of all of this—R-Day, CBT, and what is yet to come—is just not knowing. I guess this adds to the anxiety. Yet there is an air of romanticism as well. The highly regarded institution known as West Point. The Long Gray Line. Commissioned US Army officers in the making. So with the Class of 2021, another chapter is added to the continuing story.

Wait! There's a FaceTime call coming in! The adrenaline kicks in once again.

"Hi, family," Nate greets us.

"Hi, Nate," we reply as Cathy, Sam, and I sit at the kitchen table.

"Wow, Nate, look at your hair. How does it feel?" Sam asks.

Cathy and I look at Nate and we are instantly filled with joy. Such a good feeling connecting once again with our boy. Yes, our boy. I think that comment comes right out of the parent's playbook.

No matter how old our son is, knowing he has become a fine young man, he will always be our boy.

Nate has definitely thinned out; he's dropped some weight. Are they feeding him? Is he eating okay? His face looks sunken in, and it's clear to see PT and these past three weeks have had an effect on his appearance.

But Nate tells us he's doing fine. Things are busy. Early mornings. Physical training. Drilling and marching. Classroom exercises and other trainings. No shortage of things to keep these cadets occupied. Go, go, go.

Nate says that he and the other cadets will be at their sponsor's house for a few more hours, then back it is to West Point. Again, halfway through Beast and next up, A-Day!

All in all, we spend close to forty minutes chatting and FaceTiming with Nate. We got our cadet fix! Much needed. It's not been that long in real time, a few weeks. But still, the separation, the unknowns of West Point and Army life, these all add up. Yes, there's a cost, a price to pay on both sides—on the cadet and their loved ones. Not time and not money. Emotionally, there's a constant investment and then the idealistic, romantic connection to what is West Point. Mental and sweat equity. The totality of this place is profound.

Acceptance Day, or A-Day, is now less than four weeks away, August 19, 2017.

The letters continue. Nate's next update: Wednesday, July 26, 2017, 11:48 AM.

"I qualified for Land Nav! First try, yay! We had two-and-a-half hours to find 12 points on the map. The way the math works out, your total score is out of 16. To qualify, you need a 12/16 and I got a 13/16, which mean, hey, I passed! We're going back to West Point later, and we have chaplain's time tonight too! It's a good day. I'm glad I qualified on my first try."

And *The Adventures of Cadet Cody* continues too. The second volume provides a go-between with Cody's early days as our new family pet and Nate's junket to CBT.

Volume 2, July 31, 2017, captured a slew of tie-ins to a nomination letter and now Beast. "Cadet Cody: The Early Years" is all

Cody. This is the one and only edition focused entirely on one singular subject: our pooch, our treasure, our Cody. His young puppy pictures are priceless. Volume 2 shows a cadet in the making at the Canine Military Institute. There are several play on words—HRE, hands ready to eat meal, DoGMerD eye exam. The CFA, or Canine Fitness Assessment, swim test, and visions of where Cody will post someday. Lastly, a touching view of an exhausted pup after a full day of training. I think Cody can hang in there with the Class of 2021. And for the very first time, I'll admit that out of the eleven volumes writing during Nate's Plebe year, this is my *no ifs, ands, or buts* favorite. Love it!

In these short few weeks, we've already found ourselves hooked on experiencing everything that is West Point. So much so we now have plans to take in March Back on Monday, August 14. March Back is the culmination of six weeks of intense training with a twelve-mile road march from Camp Buckner to the academic post. It's the traditional end to cadet basic training and then finishes with the Acceptance Day ceremony on the Plain where the new cadets are received into the Corps of Cadets.

Cathy makes hotel reservations for an overnight stay. We'll make the trip to the academy on Sunday and get in place early Monday morning to cheer on the cadets during March Back.

Our plan is to make the six-hour trek on Sunday, August 13, and stay overnight. Get up early and stake out a place along Washington Road. But where? What time should we get there? Will Nate be able to pick us out in the crowd and see us?

Well, the good news is that Nate is thinking the very same thing. The next letter we receive from him provides the answers. He tells us that if we're coming for March Back, we should sit along the stone wall by the cemetery and fire station.

Perfect! I think.

Cathy says, "We can make signs congratulating Nate on completing Beast."

"Even better," we agree.

Cathy and I put pen to paper and get letters out to Nate, tipping him off on where we'll be and what to look for. I include a hidden gem and make myself as a harbinger. How so? I tell Nate that I'll bring the two flags, the US Flag and the West Point Flag, flying from the posts on our front porch.

"Nate, I'll stand on the cemetery stone wall and I'll be waving the flags. Keep an eye out for them! It should be easy for you to pick us out in the crowd," I tell him.

It's a perfect morning, blue sky and sunshine. Cathy, Sam, a family friend, and I pull into K-Lot above the cemetery. It's around 7:00 AM. More importantly, we beat the road closure. Washington Road is being closed to car traffic due to the new cadets, alumni, and others making their way back from Camp Buckner.

K-Lot is convenient. And part of our early arrival includes a stop at Starbucks. Caffeine is a big part of the plan. I take everyone's order and casually walk the short distance to Starbucks.

We're not quite sure when Nate will be coming through, but both sides of Washington Road are quickly filling up with proud parents, grandparents, brothers and sisters, girlfriends and boyfriends, and other loved ones. And like us, they're anxiously awaiting to see a glimpse, albeit rather briefly, of their cadet.

We stake out our section of the cemetery wall. I place my two flags along the top section, and Cathy and Sam place their poster boards against the wall.

NATO, YOU DID IT!   ★ ♥ ★

CONGRATS E-2!   ♥

BEAST IS THROUGH! Cathy has brightly colored red, white, black, and blue wording in place. Similarly, Sam has NATO, CONGRATS ON BEATING BEAST! We Love You So Much!

We have our positions!

I carry our Starbuck drinks back and take a much-welcomed drink from my grand latte. So good and much needed at this hour. I tell Cathy that I'm going to walk up and down Washington Road and check out the many varied posters in place. All pretty cool. All very touching.

Not far to the left of us, I see a poster board with E-2 Brewdawgs on it. I smile at the couple and ask if they have a cadet in E-2. They see Cathy walking toward me and ask, "Are you the Olsavskys?"

"Yes," we reply.

We quickly make our introductions and learn that Nate and their son became friends during chaplain's time. We chat for a while and exchange contact information. Our extended West Point family begins to grow.

At 7:14 AM, Cathy gets a text message. "I just got a message from a strange number," she tells us. "Maybe it's from Nate." Her face begins to beam with a smile a mile long! "It's Nate! It's a picture of Nate from someone!"

Wow, we think. It is really happening. Our cadet is doing well. He's showing a smile, but those eyes look tired.

At 7:38 AM, another text message. A picture of Nate, along with six other cadets, taking a break under the ski lifts at West Point's Victor Constant Ski Area. They are all smiles.

The adrenaline is kicking in! For us anyway. I'm pretty sure Nate and the other cadets are running on fumes at this point.

A few minutes after 10:00 AM and farther up along Washington Road, we begin to hear chants. This is soon followed by clapping, cheering, and further excitement. The Class of 2021, full rucksacks on their backs, goggles and helmets in place, make their appearance. People up and down on both sides of Washington Road are clapping, smiling, cheering, hollering.

What a magnificent, heartwarming sight to see. Sam has his tripod set up and is recording the moment. Cathy has her camera in hand, and pictures are rattling off.

The two Nate-O (NATO) poster boards are in full view, and I'm standing on top the cemetery wall, one flag pole in each arm, waving the US flag and West Point flag back and forth to the smiles of the cadets themselves.

And before too long, the companies make their way in order along the roadway—A, B, C, etc. Now we're counting. This should be E-2. Sure enough, it is.

"I see Nate, I see Nate!" Sam hollers. This is what we came for—a glimpse of our new cadet, the celebration, joy, cheering, and sharing of all the emotions of March Back from Beast.

We did it. Nate did it. The Class of 2021 did it. Congratulations! So ends March Back.

And with March Back behind us, along with Nate away, more like gone, we're now left in a somewhat fractional state. A piece of our household is missing. Are we adjusting? Well, we're getting by. Cody is helping to fill the void. And there's no shortage of dog antics. Sam takes it all in stride because he knows any attention paid to Cody is less time that we're focusing on him. How else can you characterize this? Purely, a redistribution of Mom and Dad parental oversight—targets, Sam, and Cody. They continue to remain in the crosshairs. Honestly, though, I think they like the extra attention. Isn't that how it goes? A new beginning. A new journey for all of us.

And next up is A-Day.

The letters to and from continue. We send Nate the latest on our daily and weekly happenings, and he, in turn, shares stories from Beast. It warms our hearts to hear about his successes. Little by little, he is chipping away at the beast (pun intended) and all Camp Buckner has in store.

And speaking of Camp Buckner, August 9, 2017, sees the creation of volume 3 in *The Adventures of Cadet Cody*, "Camp Barkner." We send Nate some playful pictures of Cody, Stella, and Remi in full training mode.

I can't quite remember when, but Nate later goes on to tell us that the Camp Barkner stories really lifted his spirits. I'm glad. That was the goal all along.

Sedgwick Statue. This will be our go-to meeting place following the ceremony on the Plain for Acceptance Day. Nate tells us to meet at Sedgwick in one of his final letters before A-Day. Likewise, we fill him in on our overall plans.

"Nate, we'll be coming up on Friday!" I say. "I think we'll get a chance to see you in Ike Hall. The *Black Angels over Tuskegee* Off-Broadway show is open to the public—for free."

In honor of Lt. Gen. Benjamin O. Davis Jr., the Class of 2021 will be entertained for an evening to the winner of the 2009 NAACP Award for Best Ensemble and 2009 Hollywood Artistic Director Achievement Award for Best Play.

The *Black Angels over Tuskegee* is the story of the Tuskegee airmen told in narrative of six men embarking on a journey to become pilots in the United States Army Air Forces. The play reaches deep into their collective setbacks, racial struggles with a Jim Crow mindset, their intelligence, brilliance, perseverance, and far-reaching patriotism. What an opportunity not only for Nate and his fellow cadets but for us as well.

The performance ties to the opening of Davis Barracks at West Point, aptly named in honor of Lt. Gen. Davis who passed away in 2002 at the age of eighty-nine. Davis entered West Point in 1932 as the academy's only African American cadet and was shunned during his four-year enrollment. He went on to graduate, through much adversity, and had a decorated career commanding the all-black 332nd Fighter Group, known as the Red Tails, and becoming the first black general of the United States Air Force.

Maybe Nate will be lucky enough to get assigned to Davis Barracks. Now wouldn't that be pretty cool? First year at USMA and land a gig at the brand-new facility, new latrines, showers, air-conditioning, laundry areas, office areas, etc.

Well, a post note. Perhaps I'm getting ahead of myself and the story. But as luck, or misfortune, would have it, Bradley Barracks will be Nate's new accommodations.

Pap, Cathy's dad, makes the trip to West Point with us this time. He's definitely a proud grandparent and anxious to see Nate, along with everything else associated with the academy.

We encountered heavy torrential rains along the way. From Somerset to Scranton, I had my wiper blades on max. At least the weather broke for the final stretch into New York and the last few miles to Highland Falls.

We hurriedly eat and make our way through an evening dinner at Schade's Restaurant. The Tuskegee airmen show at Eisenhower Hall starts at 7:00 PM. A free Broadway show. That doesn't come one's way that often. We pass through Thayer Gates, and I drop our party off in front of Ike Hall. I circle back and park the car at Clinton Field parking lot. I make a brisk walk, more of a fast-paced skip, back to Ike Hall.

I envision a packed auditorium. It's A-Day weekend. A free Broadway performance. Hard to pass up.

A few minutes before 7:00 PM and I open the rear left door to enter the auditorium. And to my surprise, plenty of seats. *What?* I think to myself. Crazy. Oh well. I easily find Cathy seated in the left section of the hall. More good news. Nate is standing up, up front and close to the stage, looking back and waving at us. How exciting! He tells us the new cadets were allowed to bring their phones.

The performance begins and captivates the entirety of everyone in attendance. Action, drama, history, and push-ups. So many push-ups. And like so many other great performances, the first intermission is upon us. Anyway, I let Cathy know I need to make a trip to the men's restroom, and maybe, just maybe, I'll run into Nate.

Jackpot! Walking to the restroom is Nate. I shake his hand, give him a subtle, gentle nudge, and hold back on an all-out hug. He's just as excited as I am. We chat for about a minute and he finds his way back to his seat.

With a huge smile on my face, I tell Cathy I saw Nate and talked with him. "How is he? What did he say?" she asks.

It's clear to see that he's lost some weight. His face has a sunken, hollowed look to it. And his waist is completely gone. I guess this is what six weeks of CBT Beast will do to a young vibrant body. All good though. Most importantly, he's in good spirits. Smiling, laughing, and upbeat. Yes, oh yeah, he's made it.

The *Black Angels over Tuskegee* finishes. A wonderful show. And to our delight, several of the Red Tail Airmen are here. A perfect ending. A warm, gracious, appreciative, and thankful applause fills Ike Hall.

Our exit out of Ike is entertaining also. The varied companies of new cadets rise from their seats full of energy. Plenty of smiles, their voices are reverberating through the auditorium, sounding within the open hallway, and echoing out toward the First-Class Club and Trophy Point. Everything is a competition to these kids. I can't help calling these phenomenal young men and women *kids*. Perhaps I'm just showing my age. But we clearly know they are not kids in the true sense of the word.

The cadets find different inflections and intonations—all unique to their respective companies. E is barking at something only to be responded to and more loudly by D and others. All of West Point is wrapped in a heavy late-evening fog, dampening the sounds. The sounds gradually faded, the growing blanket of heavy white fog wrapped around Ike Hall and swallowed the landscape surrounding, swooping, and indiscriminately swallowing all the buildings and trees.

The evening comes to an end.

Tomorrow is A-Day!

CHAPTER 4

Yay Day

"HI, MOM. JACOB and I made it. We're here. We hit a lot of traffic on I-81, outside of Harrisburg," Hillary tells Cathy.

"How's your Airbnb?" Cathy asks.

"It's really nice," Hillary replies. "And we're only ten minutes away from you."

"Great!" Cathy says. "I'll send you a message about meeting up in the morning when we finalize our plans here."

"Okay," Hillary says. "Good night and see you soon. I'm so excited to see Nate!"

"Love you, Hill. Good night," Cathy ends.

This weekend, to celebrate Acceptance Day at West Point, finds us staying in Cornwall-on-Hudson, a riverfront village in the town of Cornwall, Orange County, New York. A three-bedroom rental house will be our rest-and-relaxation, go-to place after we pick up Nate. Hotel accommodations, Airbnbs, resorts, etc., are all at a premium for West Point occasions such as A-Day. Cathy came through once again. A great choice and excellent find for our weekend accommodation! The house is spacious, with living room and dining room areas, laundry room, and front porch. There's plenty of room for everyone to spread out, and we can each take our turn catching up with Nate in conversations in between his naps, I'm sure.

Falling asleep comes easily. Friday finds us traveling, dining, watching a great performance at Ike Hall, sharing our adrenaline-filled excitement, and turning our thoughts to Saturday. And now it's here.

Cathy leans into me with a beaming smile. It's here, A-Day! Yay! I get to see my boy today! Early Saturday morning, we're fortunate enough to have breakfast plans at the Herbert Alumni Center sponsored by the West Point Associates of Graduates. A simple, straightforward RSVP on WPAOG website and we have our A-Day morning breakfast plans set.

On top of our breakfast arrangements is an added bonus. The first fifty people to RSVP to the WPAOG A-Day parade request receive reserved seating. Score! We made the top fifty! Good news and some not-so-good news. The allotment is only for two seats. The rest of our entourage will have to battle the crowds. Just as the oath ceremony on R-Day, the bleachers will be packed solid. Those cadets draw in the crowds!

At 7:00 AM, the cell phone rings. "Good morning, Mom," Hillary says as Cathy answers her phone.

"Hello, sweetheart," Cathy responds, followed by "Where are you? What are you up to?"

"Jacob and I are on our way to the Plain," Hillary answers back. "We'll lay out some blankets and save seats on the bleachers. We have coffee and bottled water. Would you mind bringing us something to eat? Maybe a blueberry muffin or bagel please?" she asks.

"Sure. Is there anything else you'd like?" Cathy says.

"Nope. See you soon. I'm so excited! Love you," Hillary adds.

We bypass parking at Buffalo Soldier Field to avoid riding the shuttle buses and decide to take our chances at finding a spot at the Herbert Alumni Center. Our drive along Mills Road is uneventful—a few cars, traffic is light, and we find a partially filled lot at the alumni center. We're in luck.

The WPAOG has a nice breakfast assortment set up in the dining area—coffee, tea, juice, muffins, bagels, doughnuts, fruit, and other items. We navigate our way to the reception table, make our introductions, and spot an open table. Yes! I take a seat and claim the table with our belongings. I tell Cathy and the others to get a plate of food and I'll sit and watch our stuff. I also do some people watching. There is definitely excitement and adrenaline in the air. Smiles, laughter, hugs, conversation, and many pleasantries fill the room.

Several of the old grads from the West Point Class of 1971 mingle among the crowd. They are part of the fifty-year affiliate class, with their motto: "1971 Professionally Done."

The Class of 2021 motto unveiling took place earlier in the week during March Back. Coming directly from the West Point AOG organization, the fifty-year affiliate class "1971 Professionally Done" was part of the inspiration for the design behind their crest. The simplicity yet timeless design of the Class of '71 crest is represented in the design of the 2021's crest and motto, "Until the Battle is Won."

In addition, the horizontal banner that contains the motto "Until the Battle is Won" in our crest is reflective of the horizontal banner in the 1971 crest. The Class of 2021 is the first class to have Davis Barracks in photographs of West Point. This year, Davis Barracks was opened and named after Lt. Gen. Benjamin O. Davis Jr., who graduated West Point in 1936.

To honor his legacy, on the head of the eagle are thirty-six distinct feathers to represent Davis's graduation year. Throughout the extensive design process, cadets expressed their desire to include elements of the crest that relate back to the events of 9/11 because the Class of 2021 will graduate twenty years after 9/11. On the crest, displayed are nine stars and eleven stripes on the flag. Included in the hilt of the cadet saber are seventeen lines that represent seventeen different branches of the Army that cadets will have the privilege to join upon graduation.

We are flying high this morning. Perhaps that first cup of coffee is helping us along, but I'm 110 percent certain everyone here at the AOG Center, like us, are overjoyed, ecstatic, and thrilled knowing that, in a few hours, we'll all be surrounding, hugging, and kissing our beloved Plebes. Yes, Plebes!

R-Day has come and gone, it's almost a fleeting memory now. And now, now we find ourselves within reach of Acceptance Day at West Point for our Class of 2021 sons and daughters.

The focus of A-Day is to welcome the Plebe class into the Corps of Cadets. Since R-Day, the new cadets have gone through a demanding, strenuous, and exhausting six weeks of cadet basic training. And this past Monday, we were honored to take in March Back. This is the traditional ending of CBT culminating with the twelve-mile march from Camp Buckner to the grounds of West Point. Today, we are here to celebrate and honor the newest members of the Long Gray Line.

We get our fill at breakfast and, as promised, leave with the two cups of coffee, orange juice, and two blueberry muffins for Hillary and Jacob.

"Hi, Hill," Cathy says as she lets Hillary know we're on our way to the Plain.

"We parked in the lot next to the baseball field. It looks like there are still open spots," Hill tells Cathy.

A quick and easy exit out of the Herbert Alumni Center lot finds us circling back to Thayer Road, which turns into Cullum Road. Hillary was spot-on! Open parking spots at the Doubleday Field and Clinton Field parking lots, perfect!

Pap has eyes wide-open as we pass Thayer Hall, Jefferson Hall, a.k.a. the Cadet Library. Pap takes in all the statues and monuments. "Incredible," he says. "What is that building to the left?" he asks. "There's a statue." Good catch, Pap. He takes in Patton from the front seat of the car. The General George S. Patton Jr. bronze monument statue is located in front of the library. It was moved and placed in storage for construction of the new library. In its old position, Patton faced the Old Cadet Library. It was often joked that Patton was facing the library, with binoculars in hand, so that he might now be able to better locate the building which he notably neglected as a cadet.

I make an easy left turn into Doubleday Field parking lot and find an open spot, parking close to Cullum Road. We're here! The atmosphere is electrifying. Plenty of excitement. Huge smiling and anxious faces are everywhere.

Slowly but methodically, we walk to the bleachers. And on this August 19 morning, blue sky and warm morning sun in abundance, with dew-covered grass, we look out over the Plain toward Washington Hall. What a beautiful sight! It's 8:45 AM and it seems like the minutes refuse to pass by. But soon enough, yes, before too long, everyone here will be with their beloved Class of 2021 cadet sons and daughters.

"There's Hill and Jacob," Sam says as he spots them on the bleachers, section E.

Hillary is smiling away and gives both Cathy and me big hugs.

"Coffee and muffins as promised," I say as I hand them off to Jacob.

Still an hour to go and the bleachers are fast approaching capacity. It's nice to have seats. And dry seats at that! Hillary has two large blankets laid out. Just like going to Nate and Sam's soccer games, I think to myself, those days weren't too long ago.

But here we are, seated on bleachers overlooking the Plain at the US Military Academy at West Point with a southwesterly view toward the well-maintained grass on the parade field. Washington Statue and the apron in front of Washington Hall captivate us. The sense of pride has turned into suspense and apprehension, not necessarily that something bad might happen, but more so in the sense of how these six weeks of military training have affected our new cadets. Will our son be returned to us unchanged?

And just like clockwork, 10:00 AM, Acceptance Day commences.

A cadet in the red sash has been busy attending the podium, standing directly between the review stand and the reviewing party (usually consisting of the USMA superintendent and other West Point leaders); he speaks firmly into the microphone.

The Plain is now in full display with the Hellcats and the West Point Band. The Hellcats buglers sounded attention, which alerted the cadets in the sally ports of Washington Hall that the march on is about to begin. The march on sends the cadets pouring out of the sally ports in company formation as they move in scripted fashion to their positions in the manicured grass.

The Firstie at the podium provides a narrative about the history of what will be observed in the review. He goes on to tell us about the long-standing military tradition dating back to Baron Von Steuben whose training techniques were used during the American Revolution in 1778. The goal was to create a model company, and one of the ways to do this was through drill and ceremony. Upon Von Steuben's arrival at Valley Forge, Washington's troops were far from disciplined until Von Steuben was through with them. He developed what is known as Regulations for the Orders and Discipline of the Troops of the United States of America, also known as the Blue Book.

Faint glimmers of white begin to appear in the distant sally ports. The numbers grow. An orderly procession of white and gray, in cadence, make their way onto the Plain. Families begin to identify their cadets. "I see him," we hear. "There she is!" announces someone else. Elsewhere throughout the bleachers, I witness eyes being wiped. I take my glasses off, pull a Kleenex from my pocket, and do the same. The sight of these young men and women marching in front of us penetrates our hearts and souls. It's an orchestral presentation made up of human musical notes—the various instruments, notes, and chords represented by the cadre, companies, and Class of 2021 new cadets. Unfolding before the five thousand plus in attendance on the grounds of the United States Military Academy, these sights and sounds will forever be etched in our memories.

The Corps of Cadets is divided into four regiments, each containing three battalions of three companies. Tall yellow and gray *spears* are lined up in front of us. These are the guidons. Each company has two guidons. The dress guidons displays the regimental number and the company letter above and below the initials USCC. The field guidon just has the regimental number. The colors are officially described as golden yellow and silver gray.

We have our eyes set on 2USCCE guidon, or the Second Regiment E Company. Nate is assigned to E-2, the Brewdawgs. Somewhere, standing at attention, directly in front of us, our cadet! What a sight!

It's time! The Class of 2021 new cadets, having successfully completed the grueling six and a half weeks of cadet basic training, hear the order, "New cadets, join your company."

Nate and the other cadets marched in formation into their companies and then marched past the reviewing party to the order of "Eyes right." The reviewing party includes dean of the academic board, commandant of cadets, USCC command sergeant major, USMA command sergeant major, and the superintendent of West Point.

Once past the reviewing party, each company was dismissed and continued marching back to the sally ports of Washington Hall from where they came.

After the last company has marched past, there was an announcement for the playing of the Army song, "The Army Goes Rolling Along."

There's plenty of singing from the bleachers too. Tons of smiles and conversation and overtures of where to meet. In tune, out of tune, no worries. We're set. All planned ahead. The Acceptance Day parade is completed. Next up, a short walk over to Sedgewick Statue where we will meet Nate.

Lastly, the Firstie at the podium announces an extra bonus for us. He instructs the audience to look skyward for the West Point Parachute Team. Cool! Essentially the team is trained to perform parachute demonstrations before the Army Black Knight football games and military parades at the academy. And today, the jumpers have perfect weather on a perfect day.

"Ladies and gentlemen, we have six chute canopies in the air," he calls out.

One by one, the parachutists are introduced. We follow their smoke trail and watch in amazement as they land within several feet of the landing target. The last cadet jumper, from Pittsburgh, Pennsylvania, carries the US flag in, making his 1,211th jump before the enthusiastic crowd. Wow!

The bleachers begin to quickly empty with everyone heading out into different directions. Organized chaos. Cheerful, uplifting, and high-spirited disarray, if you will. It's pretty neat just to people watch. Where do we go? Heads are turning this way and that way. Phones are out, fingers pointing everywhere. The crowds are hurriedly and decidedly on their way. In a flash, less than one hundred yards away is our predetermined rendezvous location—Sedgewick Statue.

"Nate just sent a text!" Cathy exclaims. "Let's go!"

Yeah, I think it's safe to say she's just a little bit beside herself to see her boy.

Slowly but surely, we stroll over along the sidewalk and grass, keeping pace with Pap. His knees have been giving him some problems, so we proceed at a more leisurely rate.

But in a matter of minutes, we're here! Surrounding us are numerous reunions well underway. Kisses and hugs and pictures galore.

And then, finally, Nate is walking toward us. A hero's welcoming begins.

Cathy embraces Nate, tears streaming down her cheeks as she holds on in a motherly bear hug. We all take turns greeting Nate, hugging and kissing his cheek and forehead and rubbing his shaved head. It's almost impossible not to run our hands across his bald, lockless, no-curl hair. What a difference from R-Day, going in with a full head of curly, wavy hair.

And there are differences. Nate is markedly thinner. *Holy cow*, I think. How much weight did he lose during Beast? His face has a hollowed, sunken look to it. After patting him on the back, I come to believe there isn't one bit of body fat to be found. No worries whatsoever though. He's absolutely thrilled to be with us. What a smile! A tired smile to be sure. Nate's emotions cut across the spectrum of excitement, relief, and deliverance. He doesn't seem to be alone. Looking around, the other cadets appear to be cloaked with these very same things.

A picture in front of the Sedgewick Statue is taken! What a sight! This picture will find its way to our local newspaper, the *Daily American*, Somerset County's newspaper, in a few weeks. The September 8, 2017, edition shows "With the Colors, Olsavsky Completes Training." Very proud to say the least. This same picture is posted on the Sergeant First Class Raymond Buchan Memorial Scholarship website as well. Nate was a 2017 scholarship recipient for this award given to graduating seniors in several surrounding school districts. Qualifications included having a parent, grandparent, or sibling who has honorarily served in the military or if the student has signed an obligation to serve. The scholarship honors Army Sergeant First Class Raymond Buchan of Johnstown, Pennsylvania, who was assigned to the First Battalion, Eighteenth Infantry Regiment, Second Brigade Combat Team, First Infantry Division, Schwein Fort, Germany, who died July 1, 2017, in Ta'meem, Iraq, of wounds sustained from enemy small arms fire, serving his second tour of duty in Iraq. In May of 2020, we are proud to hear that Sam is a 2020 scholarship recipient as well, making him and Nate the first siblings to be honored as such with this award. Truly humbling.

And speaking of other things, Nate has two black backpacks and one large green duffel bag. Undoubtedly packed solid with laundry. Oh yes, laundry will be on the list of things to do. Fortunately, our rental house in Cornwall has a washer and dryer. So we're in business.

We get our photo-op moments taken care of. A picture of Nate standing by the aged patina-glossed statue of Major General John Sedgwick. White over gray uniform, Olsavsky name tag, shiny brass belt buckle, and West Point cadet service cap with glowing hat badge—an Army officer in the making! A few more clicks and we toss Nate's belongings in the back of the car.

"Are we ready to leave?" I ask.

"Sure." Everyone sounds out in agreement. We decide to split into two groups. Cathy, Pap, and I will ride together and pick up pizza for lunch. Nate and the rest of the family will drive directly back to the rental house. We close the car doors and depart the parking lot.

Nate and the others plug in the address to Cornwall and are on their way. He's anxious to get out of his uniform, take a shower, put on shorts and a T-shirt, or civvies, and decompress outside of the austere confines of West Point. After six-plus weeks of nonstop physical and mental hurdles, who can blame him?

We place an order for a few tossed garden salads, antipasti salads, and three pizzas—cheese, pepperoni, and a supreme. Time to fatten Nate up! As it turns out, he dropped about fifteen pounds over the course of Beast. Funny, though, because he told us some other cadets actually gained weight. Go figure. It just goes to show how different everyone actually is. No matter, Nate is with family, and this weekend is all his.

The pickup is complete from Prima Pizza in Cornwall, and we enter the house with our hands full.

"Wow," Nate says. "That smells so good!"

He's out of his uniform and ready for lunch. Refreshed and awake, but still a bit subdued. This doesn't come as a surprise. Other West Point parents have told us that our cadet will be different when you get them back on A-Day. Amazing to see the changes from July. I see an even more mature, physically stronger, disciplined, and dynamic young man. Nate isn't the same person we dropped off and whom we said our sixty-second goodbyes to on R-Day. The depth of pride, the layers of gratitude, and a growing indebtedness are reaching deep inside not only Cathy and me but to our family and friends. It means something much more when I overhear someone say, "Thank you for your service" to our service members.

Everyone has their fill of pizza. Thumbs-up to Prima Pizza! We have the kitchen stocked up with an assortment of snacks: potato chips, pretzels, candy, cookies, and fresh fruits of watermelon, strawberries, blueberries, and oranges.

Nate is undeniably the center of attention.

"Nate, can I get you something to drink?" Cathy asks. "Do you want some chocolate chip cookies? Everything is on the counter here, so just help yourself," she tells everyone.

Each of us take turns talking to Nate, asking him questions, but making sure we don't inundate him with our barrage of inquiries. We try to avoid the cross-examination in our overzealous efforts to pick Nate's memory. We're trying to piece together the six-week information gap. Just a thirst of sorts to fill in the time gap. All in its due course, it will come together.

Nate has his laptop out and is checking e-mails on his class schedule. Several of his instructors have already sent out their course syllabuses. Monday is the start of classes. And the next step in his forty-seven-month journey to commissioning. But up next is something much simpler and more pressing—a nap. We figured he'd need his rest.

"I'm going upstairs to lie down," Nate tells us. "I'm exhausted. Wake me up in an hour," he says as he walks toward the stairs.

Cathy gives him a kiss on the forehead as he passes by. A silent glow of motherly love. This scene is undoubtedly being played out countless times elsewhere throughout the Hudson Valley.

Up next, laundry! Lots of laundry. Three full bags to be exact. And what catches our eyes? Of all things, the large safety pins. These are net laundry bag pins, five inches long, to be used for a variety of functions. But now, we just need to get them threaded out and looped off the bag strings. Mission accomplished! The first load of Nate's dirty West Point clothing is in the washer.

Since R-Day, we've been wondering what became of Nate's clothes he wore that morning—socks, shorts, and his green Under Armor Army shirt. Well, we have our answer. Rolled up in a quart-sized Ziploc bag are Nate's clothes. And the $64,000 question: what aroma awaits us when we open the bag? Yikes! Uh, nothing. Not bad at all. No different than Nate's pile of laundry in his room from high school. Whew, what a relief. His R-Day clothes make their way into the next load of laundry. One load in and out. Progressing nicely. We're admiring his white shirts, gray slacks, ACUs (Army combat uniform), and socks. Plenty of socks and T-shirts too. All being washed. And now fresh, clean, and folded.

Nate saunters down the stairs and is welcomed to a resounding "Hi, Nate" from everyone. Easy to see that he enjoyed his nap. He's getting his sleep deprivation satisfied in lockstep with his appetite.

Nate plops down at the kitchen table and turns to his laptop to once again check his e-mails, schedule, and class supply list. It looks like we'll be making a trip to Walmart after dinner to pick up first-day-of-school supplies. Unlike the beginning of the 2016–2017 school year last September, Nate will soon be provided a focused academic, military, and physical instruction regimen in the most elite moral-ethical environment in the world. Yes, two days away.

The afternoon is passing at breakneck speed, and we're already talking about dinner. We have reservations at Schlesinger's Steak House in new Windsor. A night out with our cadet! Proud, excited, and elated. Our emotions are beyond words.

For A-Day weekend, Plebes must wear their uniforms while they are out in public. This mandatory uniform requirement can change year to year, but for the Class of 2021 cadets, it's a "wear your uniform at all times when out in public." Like us, other families will be parading their uniformed Plebes out and about as they make the journey for dinner or school items or simply to spend time away from their lodgings. All within a seventy-five-mile radius of West Point though. Plebes are restricted to this distance and must report back to West Point by taps on Saturday evening and must return back to the barracks on Sunday for accountability at 7:00 PM.

My maps app is showing a little over eight miles and ten minutes to Schlesinger's Steak House from our Airbnb. But we know better. These serpentine roads within the Hudson Valley cut through a various series of rock types and make for interesting roadways and driving. Intriguing and gripping, yes, not so agreeable for passengers in the back seat who are prone to car sickness.

Nonetheless, we arrive at Schlesinger's. An uneventful drive. The parking lot is full, but fortunately, we have reservations. Everything for this weekend has been methodically and meticulously planned by Cathy. We're progressing through our to-do checklist like a well-oiled machine.

Like Nate, several other cadets are adorned with their white-over-gray uniforms and hats delicately placed underneath or beside them and their families. Smiles and warm conversation are in plentiful supply.

Admittedly, the atmosphere and environment on this A-Day evening is raising eyebrows. It's hot and humid outside, but the wide French-style doors are opened widely on the side wall. So much for a cool, air-conditioned, overly comfortable setting. Nonetheless, being with Nate and enjoying a steak dinner makes up for our minor gripes—with one exception. I asked our waiter for A-1 steak sauce for my marbled rib eye. Big mistake! I received an elite lecture that the pure, extravagant flavor of these beef cuts do not require accompaniments of any kind—no ifs, ands, or buts. I pressed on and reluctantly the waiter acquiesced to me. I went on to thoroughly enjoy my steak while dipping bite-size pieces of tasty steak into my A-1. A memory was made.

There is still a look of tiredness on Nate's face as we engage in conversation and eat our meals. It's different than when we first met him at Sedgewick. I think his energy level was still on the decline at that point. But now, while drained and somewhat burned out, his batteries are recharging. He's on the upswing. So good to see. It seems like similar scenes are being played out at the other tables in the restaurant. Looks of delight, laughter, smiles, pats on the back, and cadet rejuvenation. These A-Day memories will forever connect the Class of 2021 families and friends.

Well, our attention now turns to Nate's school supplies checklist. Cathy and I volunteer to make a trip to Walmart and Staples to pick up notebooks, paper, paper clips, Post-it notes, pens, pencils, stapler, staples, cleaning supplies, coffeepot, etc. But not before another photo-op moment! We line up in front of the entranceway to Schlesinger's and as perfect timing would have it, a courteous young lady offers to take our picture. Snap!

Our two groups part ways. Cathy and I head to Walmart and everyone else make their way back to the house. Nate can relax and kick back in comfort and catch up with everyone, then go shopping. No argument on that front. Our boy is back in his element, eating and sampling everything in sight, surfing on his iPhone, catching up with friends, and getting us up to speed on his last six weeks. So nice!

I pull into the parking lot at the Walmart in Newburgh, New York, and not surprisingly, the identical matter in hand is being played out—cadets in their white-over-gray uniforms, side by side with their moms and others, entering and exiting the store, carrying multiple bags. Notebooks, binders, Swiffer Sweepers and sweeping pads, Clorox wipes, coffeepots, and the list goes on. It's our turn now.

Slowly but surely, the shopping cart is being filled. And then as we second-guess what Nate may need, and as luck would have it, Cathy overhears a cadet talking with his father and sees that he is looking at a supply list that was sent to all cadets. What? Nate didn't say anything about this!

"Excuse me," Cathy introduces herself and explains that she has a son at West Point. She politely asks the handsome young cadet if he would mind sharing his supply list with her.

"Yes, ma'am, sure," he enthusiastically replies. "We were e-mailed a list of items," he goes on to say. He then sent Cathy a pic of the list. I guess Nate is behind on e-mails. No matter. We pick up everything and a few extra items. Mission accomplished. Pretty cool to hear "Yes, ma'am," "Thank you, sir," and other courteous, polite niceties when encountering these fine young men and women.

"Wow, thank you, guys," Nate tells us with a beaming smile as we carry the Walmart bags in through the front door to the table where he is seated in front of his laptop. He takes a look at everything, bag by bag, as if it's Christmas morning. "Thank you again," he says.

Snacking, making catch-up conversation, watching TV, and folding laundry fill in the remainder of this Saturday A-Day evening, Nate, or for that matter, all of us, are getting a long overdue dose of vitamin F(amily). And it's working.

I can't help but think of the letter Nate sent us a few weeks ago. He told us that he had a few letters and was reading them among his two Beast roommates.

"Hey, Olsavsky, that must be some letter," his roommate says as a flow of tears begin to make their tracks down Nate's cheeks.

"Yeah," Nate responds back to him. "Just reading about everything back home. A little homesick."

A few extra prayers and warm thoughts are sent Nate's way after reading his letter. That type of raw, pure emotional candor really tugs deep into our hearts. That's what love is, that's what love does.

Nate is tired, we are tired, everyone is tired. A lot has been packed in today. Nate is battling to keep his eyes open. It is 10:30 PM.

"What do you think, Nate?" Cathy asks while she simultaneously answers the question. "Let's get you back to post and you can text us when you want us to pick you up in the morning."

Nate is worn out and beyond drowsy, and with eyes half closed, he agrees, "Yeah, let's head back."

The others in the house easily find the inside of their eyelids this Saturday night as we depart. Tomorrow is another day.

Pap beats everyone as the first to get moving this Sunday morning. A quiet, tranquil view from the front porch looking out across the railroad tracks and onto the fast-moving Hudson River. We've gotten used to the steady flow of train traffic coming through and are unaffected—pure tiredness. Everyone sleeps through the periodic rumbling of the engines and railcars passing by.

But on this early morning, a new guest joins our family. Or should I say Pap has a newfound friend, a gray feline who has joined him for his morning cup of coffee on the porch? A neighborhood gray tabby cat perhaps. By the looks of it, though, you'd think Pap and his gray-and-white-striped smoke-colored guest have been "rise and shine coffee-drinking" partners forever. Too funny.

"Pap, what are you doing?" Cathy protectively asks. "That cat could be a stray and have rabies! Be careful you don't get scratched or bitten!"

I think she has visions that Pap will somehow end up as an episode on *Animal Planet*'s "Monsters Inside Me" television series. Part horror movie, part medical detective story. This show depicts what happens when people fall prey to an infection from a parasite or some other nasty microscopic creature.

Pap calmly replies, "Don't worry, he's a neighborhood cat" as he laughs off concern.

Sam and I take in the drama and almost, hand in hand, think the same thing. "Pap, what would Cody do if he saw you with that cat?" Never a dull moment.

Now Sunday, a day of worship, we travel nearby to St. Patrick's Catholic Church in Newburgh, New York, for 10:30 AM Mass. Our weekend is winding down. It is only a matter of hours, not days, before Nate reports back and preps for the start of his Plebe academic year. This warm, sunny morning is perfect, though, and like us, there are other West Point families with their Plebes giving thanks at St. Patrick's.

It's easy to spot the white shirts over gray pants along with brand new hats closely guarded in the church pews. New cadets giving thanks, collectively in prayer, with all in attendance this morning. Love of God, country, and family—these young men and women have their priorities in order.

Lunchtime. Out trek finds us on a path back to leftovers: salad, pizza, wings, fruit, and all the other goodies we brought along for the weekend. There's plenty of food to choose from, and better yet, we're in the quiet, comfortable atmosphere of the rental and a lot of upbeat, cheerful conversation. Talk ensues around the start of classes and trying out for the club soccer team. His first academic week will be busy!

"Take care and love you bunches," Hillary tells Nate in the middle of a humongous sisterly hug. She plants a goodbye kiss on his head as well.

"You'll do great, Nate-O. We're so proud of you!"

She and Jacob say their goodbyes to Pap, and the rest of us and get on their way back home to Chambersburg.

"Safe travels, love you," Cathy tells Hill. "Let us know when you get home."

Where is our time machine? I wonder. I want to hit a reset button, but that's just wishful thinking.

"You will never have this day with your children again. Tomorrow, they'll be a little older than they were today. This day is a gift. Breathe and notice. Smell and touch them. Study their faces and little feet and pay attention" (unknown).

Yes, these past several days, Cathy and I have done exactly this. We realize Nate is older, more mature, a young man, an American soldier. He is a gift that we cherish. How many times did I run my hand over his shaved head? How many times did Cathy hug and kiss him on the forehead and cheek? We've studied our young son up and down and sideways.

Like grains of sand passing through the metaphorical hourglass, our sands of time have run out. This A-Day weekend has come and gone, and Nate is due back for accountability in a few hours.

Let's make the most of this time and see one more thing. Cathy is the planner extraordinaire in this regard.

"There's a path and boat docks along the Hudson," she says. "We can stop along the way and enjoy some of the sights."

No argument from anyone to savor the remaining time with Nate. Another gorgeous day; sunshine, warm temps, and blue sky complete the picture. And speaking of picturesque, the view from the docks out along the Hudson is captured by Cathy. *Click, click, click.* Nate is front and center in each pic. So nice! But all good things must come to an end. I've lost count on how many times we've traveled back and forth on the zigzag roadways to West Point. The Tuskegee airman led the opening curtain call for A-Day weekend, and the final curtain call has us showing our IDs to the security guards at Thayer Gate.

A different set of identifications pass us by along Thayer Road as we head to Grant Hall turnaround. License plates from Georgia, New Hampshire, Missouri, North Carolina, and elsewhere reflect the fabric of the common bond, cadets, and their families from all walks of life, linking us together in the Long Gray Line.

And together we are! Together in saying our goodbyes. Together in familiarity with hugs and kisses and tears. Clean laundry, school supplies, coffeepots, and cleaning items are plentiful. Walmart bags and the sort are being pulled out of the rear of cars.

I put the car in park and pop open the rear hatch. Everyone exits the car. This send-off is markedly different compared to the July 2 R-Day goodbyes. Another new beginning in Nate's West Point journey.

What an exciting week this has been for Nate and the other Class of 2021 cadets. After completing CBT, they found themselves in the midst of yet another challenging experience—Reorganization Week (a.k.a. Reorgy Week). They are scrambled from their CBT companies into their academic-year companies and find themselves with new roommates. They were issued their phones and now are reconnected with the outside world. Hurry up and wait has been the order of business for most of the week. Right back to standing in lines. Being issued their computers and printers and textbooks. Their virtual mailboxes are already full of messages about assignments from their professors that are due on the first day of classes. But success comes one step at a time.

I try my best not to cry but fail miserably. Salty tracks of tears are not in short supply with our send-off. Looking at others in Grant turnaround and across from the admission building, the very same scenes are being played out. Lots of tears. Joyful tears, albeit in abundance. Tears of love and pride and infinite caring.

Nate is strapped with his green laundry bag, backpack, and supplies.

What is running through Nate's mind? I pause to wonder. With our final hugs, pats on the back, kisses, and well wishes, Nate walks away down past the guard post and, step-by-step, fades away down the sidewalks into the humbling architecture of West Point.

Soft, gentle, quiet whispers of "Love you, Nate" and we proceed to get back into the car. Other families are awaiting their turn.

"Bye, Nate."

So much history, so many things to take in on these impressive USMA grounds. Pap is interested in seeing some of the West Point sights. Onto Williams Road and we pass the Class of '47 old train station adjacent to the south dock. Up and over the hillside, back toward Thayer Hall along Cullum Road, we look across the Plain and toward Trophy Point on the right. A turn onto Stoney Lonesome Road leads us to Lusk Reservoir and Michie Stadium with few words spoken. Pretty cool, though, all the history along with the stories. I slowly drive along Washington Road and we decide to stop and tour the cemetery.

The very sacredness of these time-honored grounds sends a chill up my spine. The West Point cemetery holds within its gates memorials to some of America's most storied military leaders and historic figures including Bvt. Brigadier General Sylvanus Thayer, General Norman Schwarzkopf, Major General Daniel Butterfield, and Lieutenant Colonel George Custer, along with other notable heroes, astronauts, and eighteen Medal of Honor recipients.

A fitting end to our A-Day celebration and weekend with our cadet, Nate, who, right at this minute, is settling in to Bradley Barracks with Company E-2, the Brewdawgs, and his new roommates.

Monday morning, August 21, 2017, and Cornwall-on-the-Hudson is in our rearview mirror. What would the first day of school be without a first day of school picture? Nate delivers. And Cathy is thrilled. Gray slacks, a black short-sleeve shirt with his nameplate, and gray-black hat with shield. What an amazing picture! He didn't forget to send mom a pic.

Driving along Interstate 84, we leave New York and enter Pennsylvania. For whatever reason, Sam gets a kick out of passing through this area, particularly Matamoras. It is the easternmost municipality of any kind in Pennsylvania and located at the tristate border of New York, New Jersey, and Pennsylvania. Go figure.

Besides Sam's unusual affinity for Matamoras, today is a very special day for another reason. The great American eclipse will be visible anywhere in the mainland United States. And the weather is cooperating. The sky is relatively clear, just a few clouds lingering as we travel along I-80 and approach I-99/220 near Penn State's University Park main campus.

Both sunroof panels are open in our Ford Explorer, so we have full view above us. At 2:34 PM, it begins. We're taking in an amazing sight—a total eclipse. Something that hasn't happened since 1918. Notably, this total eclipse marked the first such event in the social media era in America. Breathtaking, amazing, and incredible. NASA stated that "never before will a celestial event be viewed by so many and explored from so many vantage points—from space, from the air, and from the ground."

Ironically, overshadowing the predictions, appearance, and viewing of the solar eclipse are our memories of Acceptance Day 2017 at the United States Military Academy at West Point for the Class of 2021.

CHAPTER 5

Weekend Pass, the Holidays, and, Oh, That Army-Navy Game Too!

THIS SUMMER OF 2017 has certainly kept us busy—Sam's recovery from surgery, Nate's departure to West Point, and moving Hillary and Jacob into their new house. What else can we possibly squeeze in before Sam heads back to school next Tuesday? Well, there is one more thing: the beach. A few days in Ocean City, Maryland. Sun, surf, sand, and seafood. A chance to just relax on the beach and work on our tans. Previous trips to Ocean City had Sam, Nate, and I timing the break in the waves with boogie boards strapped to our wrists. We'd make a competition out of each attempt to catch and ride the tumultuous waves. Without fail, yours truly would always score a perfect ten. I would unmercifully judge Sam and Nate, seeing them usually coming in with a four or five. Too funny.

This trip is different. We're down one familiar face. No Nate to accompany us and Sam is unable to tackle the waves with me. But Hillary and Jacob join us for two days, and we enjoy soaking in the high 80°F sun, walking the brightly lit boardwalk, and making our customary stop for saltwater taffy, doughnuts, fudge, and candied apples. And of course, dinner out at Phillips Seafood House for all-you-can-eat crab legs. Cathy and Sam opt for the Alaskan king crab legs this year, and I join them. Delicious!

Sam begins his sophomore year at Somerset High School, and this Tuesday, August 29, 2017, he's the lone ranger for Cathy's first day of school picture on the front porch. This will be an exciting year though. Why? Sam's learner's permit for his driver's license. Yep, come December, Sam will be driving. All part of growing up, I guess.

A-Day weekend and our brief but much-needed Ocean City, Maryland, vacation provides plenty of material to work with for Cadet Cody. The adventure volumes continue and gives Nate a boost and dose of family connection at the right times.

Nate's semester is off to a busy start. He attended tryouts for the Army Club Soccer Team and planned on trying out for an open position on the Division I Soccer Team. Perhaps a reflection of his maturity and knowing his boundaries, he passes on the D-I opportunity and goes with the club team. Not that playing D-I was a given, still nice to see his talent was recognized. Fantastic! More soccer to come. We've not seen the last of his soccer career and playing days. We check out the club team schedule and make arrangements to travel and watch two home games at West Point. Each of us seem to be finding our groove with the new family dynamics. Cody continues to entertain us; he can run up a full flight of stairs now. Sam was cleared by his orthopedic surgeon to play soccer and is making his comeback with the JV and varsity high school team. Cathy is busy keeping order to our weekly schedules and monitoring the West Point Moms' Facebook page, along with everything else West Point. And me, besides creating the next in line of *The Adventures of Cadet Cody*, I dive into reading a few books: *The Lords of Discipline* by Pat Conroy, *Brothers Forever* by Tom Manion and Tom Sileo, *Absolutely American* by David Lipsky, and *West Point 1915: Eisenhower, Bradley, and the Class the Stars Fell On* by Michael E. Askew. Easy enough to pick out the overreaching subject matter and where a good portion of my thoughts reside.

It's been almost two months since Nate last stepped out away from home departing for R-Day. Now we hear some really good news from him.

"Hi, Mom and Dad," he says. "It looks like we're going to get a free pass for Labor Day weekend! Would you guys want to pick me up so I could come home for the weekend?" he asks on the phone.

Cathy and I quizzically glance at each other and smile. Maybe more like beaming smirks, as if we would say no.

"Yes!" Cathy loudly replies.

"The opening-day Army Black Knights football game is Friday, so we can't leave until Saturday morning," he tells us. "I think we'll get released Saturday at 5:00 AM. I'll let you know for sure toward the end of the week." He ends by telling us, "Love you."

Our minds are going a million miles a minute!

"We get our boy back!" Cathy enthusiastically hollers.

The wheels are set in motion, and we discuss our options for pickup and return to West Point. The Moms' Page is abuzz, in overdrive, and collaboration messages and requests are in full swing, along the lines of "I can pick up three cadets on Saturday if someone is able to take them back on Monday."

Luckily, we're within driving distance of West Point. Cathy and I decide to make both trips—pickup on Saturday and return on Labor Day, Monday. Cathy reaches out to the Western Pennsylvania West Point Parents' Club and informs the group that we have room for one cadet.

I quickly realize what we just committed to do: two round trips in a matter of three days. Caffeine can be your best friend, lol.

Saturday morning, 5:20 AM. The time is set. Nate calls to let us know he'll get released a bit after 5:00 AM. *Released*, I think. Sounds rather harsh. As if he's getting a weekend pass away from prison. Well, with limited freedom and liberties, always being told where to be, when to be there, and accounted for, who can argue?

We'll have a full car. Six of us in total. Cathy, Sam, me, Nate, and two other cadets—a third-year cadet and a Plebe. One is the nephew of Cathy's friend, and the other responded to Cathy's parent's club message about having an open seat for a Pittsburgh area cadet looking for a ride home to the Pittsburgh area.

"Brrr, I can't believe how cold it is! It's showing 39°F," I tell Cathy and Sam as we make our first pit stop at mile 224 on I-80. The good thing is that the crisp, cold, smack-in-the-face early-morning air is a refreshing jolt to help keep me awake for the drive. It's around 1:30 AM, and we're three-plus hours away from West Point. I have my diet Mountain Dew to give me a caffeine boost. Sam is cozy in the back seat, sound asleep, while Cathy and I fill the passing miles with conversation and small talk. Where should we stop for breakfast on the way back? We both say Nate and the other cadets will probably sleep along the way back. We brought blankets and pillows for that very reason. Let's make these cadets, our kids, as comfortable as possible. They deserve it. It goes with being a part of the West Point family. Taking care of Nate, these cadets, or any other cadet is second nature. Just like being a parent. This type of caring comes naturally and is unconditional.

Mile after mile after mile, we drive on. Oddly enough, the time on the road wasn't over tiring after all. Traffic was light and the weather was good. Stars galore. It's around 4:45 AM as we make our way down the winding roads into Highland Falls. I take Cathy up on her suggestion. We park across from the Park Restaurant on Main Street in Highland Falls and recline back in our car seats. We'll make an attempt to get in a fifteen- to thirty-minute power nap. Now all that remains is to wait for a call from Nate.

Cathy's phone rings, 5:15 AM. "Hi, Mom. Where are you guys?" Nate asks. "I'm getting my bags together and I'll be on my way."

Before Nate can even get the words out of his mouth, Cathy is responding, "Good morning, Nate! How are you? We're in front of the Park Restaurant. Where should we pick you up?"

"Can you come to Grant turnaround? I'll let the others know too," Nate says.

"Sure, take your time," Cathy says. "We'll be there."

Grant turnaround is abuzz with cars and cadets. It's cold and dark outside, but the excitement is overpowering. Cadets in white-over-gray uniforms make their way past the guard post and quickly find their anxious loved ones waiting. Smiles, hugs, kisses, pats on the back are teeming.

And then Nate appears, and we join the foray in these early hours at West Point. Our other two riding companions soon appear, and we make our introductions and pack their belongings in the car. We're set!

"I bet you're excited to get away for a few days," I announce to the group.

Some muffled conversation ensues. Lack of sleep and tiredness is written all over their faces. Cathy lets them know to help themselves to the pillows and blankets and get comfy. I tell them to sneak in some shut-eye and we'll make a stop in Wilkes Barre for breakfast—Cracker Barrel. A resounding "sounds good" fills the air and we depart West Point.

Nate and Sam find their comfort zones in the rear seats while the other two in the middle seats, each leaning against the doors. Eyes are closed, heads are comfortably resting, and Cathy and I smile at each other. Pickup is complete. Next, a prayer for safe travels home.

And once again, my focus is on the road and the passing miles. Am I tired? Yes, a bit. But not exhausted. I keep telling Cathy to close her eyes and sleep, but as always, she stands in as my copilot and refuses. She'd rather keep me company and help me focus.

Funny thing, though, my thoughts are on our soon-to-be breakfast stop. I'm so looking forward to a cup of coffee (or two or three)!

The two-hour drive quickly passes by, snoozing in the back seats, along with small talk, and I take Exit 168 off I-81 and pull into the Cracker Barrell parking lot.

"Good morning again, everyone," I say. "Who's ready for breakfast?"

Yawns, leg stretches, and arms raised in the air appear as we exit the car. The smell of bacon, pancakes, coffee and seeing French toast, ham and eggs, and waffles on tables as our waitress seats us bring our three West point cadets out of their languor.

There are plenty of eyes and heads turning inside Cracker Barrel as our two Plebes walk by carrying their white hats and dressed in white over grays. Our third-year cadet, a Cow, isn't required to be in uniform when leaving the academy. Cathy and I are bursting with pride and are simply thrilled to treat Nate and his friends to a much-welcomed breakfast.

And before too long, we pull into the McDonald's parking lot near the Somerset I-76 turnpike exit and meet up our parent friends. We make our introductions, exchange a few pleasantries, along with a few hugs, and everyone departs for home. We have our cadets home and plan to make the most out of this Labor Day weekend.

Saturday comes and goes. We take our naps to catch up on some much-needed sleep and go to Rey Azteca, a local Mexican restaurant in Somerset for dinner, a favorite place of Nate's and Sam's and, admittedly, a favorite of Cathy and mine too.

Nate shares his stories of how classes are going and how he's able to balance club soccer. We're all ears and latch on to every word. He shows us his new soccer uniform and warm-up suit. Looks great! French, math, English, and chemistry courses find their way into our conversations. All good. And so glad to hear. So far, West Point looks like a positive fit for Nate.

And just like A-Day weekend, several loads of laundry are being taken care of, cleaned, sorted, and folded for our cadet. We're not complaining though. Words can't even begin to describe what it's like to have Nate back home. Cody may have been more excited than us. His little tail and butt were moving a million miles a minute when he laid eyes on Nate. How cute! And hopefully, some material to work with for a volume of Cadet Cody.

Now we find ourselves greeting Sunday morning, along with 10:00 AM Mass at St. Peter's. Nate isn't thrilled with our request. "Will you wear your uniform to Mass, Nate?" we ask. Hard to describe the looks we get back from him. A simple nah or no would have sufficed. Reluctantly, Nate agrees. He dresses up in his white over grays.

Yes, I must admit, there is an ulterior motive for our request. Call it what you will, but I'll chalk it up to joy, pride, and pure mom-and-dad love. Of course, we want to show off our West Point cadet son!

Nate undeniably sticks out—tall, handsome, shaved head, and dressed in uniform. Father O'Neill greets us as we enter the church and make our way in. A big smile ensues from Father O'Neill, along with a hug and pat on the back. He is happy that Nate is doing well. And lastly and without hesitation, almost a given, Father rubs Nate's hairless head. Too funny. Just like A-Day all over again. What is it with haircuts, especially when someone gets a bald cut? The overwhelming hankering to run your hand across their head. Who knows?

It's been a fantastic couple of days this Labor Day weekend, but all good things must come to an end. We do a sanity check on when our next opportunity to see Nate will be. Family Weekend is scheduled for October 20–22, 2017, and we plan to make the trip. Until then, Monday is upon us, and we meet our cadet passengers again at McDonald's in Somerset. We undertake the reverse travel itinerary of what we drove a few days ago—Somerset to West Point and back home. We're doing an all-day road trip again. Looking at roughly thirteen hours to and from, but all worth it. Our much-welcomed and delightful weekend is wrapped up.

Club soccer is in full swing! Nate is thoroughly enjoying the games, the competitiveness, but not so much with the impact of the practices after class and having to balance his coursework, company fall sport, and other training demands. All part of high pressure, high stress, "throw everything at the plebes" to prepare them in their journey to become US Army second lieutenants.

We agree on one phone call per week, Sunday evening, to lessen Nate's time-management burdens. We tell him that a once-a-week check-in is perfectly fine to touch base and keep us up-to-date on all his activities. The letter writing continues, as does the newer releases of Cadet Cody, and we make it perfectly clear that we're only a phone call away—any day, anywhere, any time. If you need to reach out, just call. That's our message to Nate and in many ways, I think it helps him knowing that we have his back and we're here for him when needed.

It's so exciting to hear that Nate is a starter for the club team, rotating between the defender and mid-positions. Pretty cool, and I'm sure it provides a bit of a throwback to his high school senior year season. Nate sends us pictures of his practice and game uniforms, and warm-up sweat suits and even better pictures from his first away game. A perfect opportunity to disconnect from what probably seems like the walls closing in at West Point.

The brief afternoon respite serves its purpose in several ways. The Army Black Knights notch up a win! And the return trip back to West Point finds the team making a pit stop for fast food. McDonald's it is! A win and something to eat other than what these cadets have been getting from Washington Hall. Life is good!

Yepper, life is good but insanely busy with a no-room-to-breathe schedule. Nate tells us that club soccer doesn't get him out of his commitment to participate in company athletics. So in addition to club practice, he has E-2 company soccer games mixed in as well. No shortage of soccer.

And no shortage of Cathy missing Nate terribly, so this brings in a change of plans of next seeing Nate at Family Weekend. As it turns out, Cathy, along with Hillary and some friends from home, decides to travel to see one of Nate's soccer games. So in the early hours on Saturday morning of September 16, the four of them set out on their road trip to get another dose of Nate. Who can argue? I stay behind to tend to Sam with homework, plus he's on the schedule to referee on Sunday. Sam, like Nate, is a certified soccer referee for our local traveling soccer teams program, which is part of the Western Pennsylvania Soccer Club. And similar to Nate, Sam shares his gripes when he has two games scheduled to referee rather than a one-and-done Sunday afternoon. But at the end of the season, both of our boys always lit up and enjoyed getting their paycheck. Cha ching! Payday!

The girls make it safely to the US Military Academy Preparatory School (USMAP) field and get a rare opportunity to actually see Nate in action on the field. Even better yet, the afternoon's action sees a 2–1 Army Black Knight win over the Yale Bulldogs. Go Army! Their evening is then topped off with dinner at Schade's Restaurant. Sunday morning finds the five of them enjoying a delicious breakfast at Fiddlesticks Café in Cornwall. A small, tight-seated place but the breakfast items—blueberry pancakes, omelets, eggs, bacon, etc.—are really delicious. With menu items names like On Blueberry Hill,

Benedict's Eggs, Wrapped up in Burritoville, and Humpty Dumpty Had a Great Fall, you can't go wrong! The place kind of has that diners, drive-ins, and dives type of food. And one that becomes a go-to place for us on subsequent visits to West Point.

The following Sunday, September 24, Nate gets another break from the academy grounds as a contingent of West Point cadets make their way to the Tunnels to Tower run in New York City.

On this warm, bright Sunday morning, with the changing of season right around the corner, more than half of West Point's cadets, nearly 2,400 staff, faculty, and US Military Academy Prep School personnel volunteered their time to participate in the annual Tunnel to Towers 5K Run and Walk in New York City.

The event memorializes NYC firefighter Stephen Siller, who was off duty when the planes, overtaken by Al-Qaeda terrorists, directed the flights to hit the World Trade Center on September 11, 2001. Instead of going golfing with his brothers, Siller returned to his squad to grab his firefighting equipment. He drove his truck to the Brooklyn Battery Tunnel, but it was already closed. He then strapped on sixty pounds of gear and rushed on foot through gridlocked traffic and ran, determined and unselfish, from the tunnel to the towers where he gave his life while saving others. How true are the words from the Bible, John 15:13: "No one can have greater love than to lay down his life for his friends."

This is where the lines converge between the selfless act of NYFD firefighter Stephen Siller and the West Point Corps of Cadets—duty, honor, country. This is where reality also sets in knowing that our sons and daughters are committed to place themselves in harm's way in service to God and country, family, and friends and a profound calling that has led them to the Long Gray Line. Without question, these cadets have our love, respect, caring, and thoughts and prayers.

The next four weeks fly by quickly and the October 20–22, 2017, fourth annual Family Weekend at USMA arrives. Friday morning greets us with warm, piercing sunshine and pleasant blue skies. Nate and his fellow cadets have a full class schedule. No rest or respite for the very busy Corps of Cadets. Visiting families, on the other hand, had the opportunity to join briefings, visit the library, and visit the simulation center, where Sam and Nate took turns trying to outdo each other as expert marksmen firing in the engagement skills trainer.

This is our first Family Weekend, and we're loving the chance to see Nate in uniform and watch him in the West Point environment. And we're also anxious to attend our very first Army football game—Army versus Temple. Nate then takes us into the library. Such a cool place. The USMA library has a display of academy rings. The three rings centered and highlighted in the middle of the case are those of Generals Bradley, MacArthur, and Eisenhower. Rings shown from more recent classes of the Long Gray Line belonged to those who, unfortunately and sadly, died in recent conflicts, paying the ultimate sacrifice while serving their country.

Interestingly, another tradition in the long line of traditions involving the rings has to do with the Plebes' reactions to first seeing the new rings at which time the Firsties are mobbed by Plebes reciting the "Ring Poop":

> Oh my gosh, sir/ma'am, what a beautiful ring.
> What a crass mass of brass and glass.
> What a bold mold of rolled gold.
> What a cool jewel you got from your school.
> See how it sparkles and shines.
> It must have cost you a fortune.
> Please, sir/ma'am, may I touch it?
> May I touch it please, sir/ma'am?

Next up, Nate leads us through the courtyard and walkways to meet his math instructor, who teaches MA153 mathematical modeling and introduction to differential equations, otherwise known as jedi math. The course description for MA153 is enough to send your mind racing to a galaxy far, far away; study topics include first order differential equations, Laplace transforms, series solutions techniques, and nonlinear equations and stability. Need I say more?

The instructor engages in pleasant chitchat with Cathy and me. A West Point grad himself, he tells us how exciting it is to be back as a professor and helping these cadets succeed in their forty-seven-month journey to becoming a commissioned officer. He lets us know that Nate is doing incredibly well. We can't help but be elated after hearing that.

The conversation serendipitously turns to our evening plans. Nate shares that he plays on the club soccer team and has a game at 5:30 PM on the USMAPS soccer field. As it turns out, his instructor is a soccer fan having played and spent time as the graduate assistant soccer coach at the US Military Academy Prep School, Fort Monmouth. On the spot, he tells us that it's been awhile since he's taken time to watch a game and lets us know he'll be there this evening. Pretty cool how things work out!

We make a stop in Grant Hall, located in the heart of Central Area. Grant Hall is a thriving hub of activity for cadets and faculty and others to meet, grab something to eat outside of Washington Hall, or just grab a cup of coffee and waste time. Coffee, tea, Coke, and cookies find their way to our table. No complaints. Our legs are tired and feet sore from all the walking. It's a nice break and gives us a chance to recharge.

It's difficult to pass up a trip to the gift stores. So we make our way to two stops. First, the cadet store and then the gift store on the fourth floor in Thayer Hall. A hoodie, long-sleeve shirt, ball cap, pocketknife, and a few other items make up our purchases. The stores are busy, busy, busy. And it's challenging not to pass up on the cool West Point items. I'm hooked. I could buy anything and everything West Point related, but Sam and Cathy reel me in. Good thing and even better news for my wallet.

It's Friday evening, and we find our way to the USMAPS field. We spot Nate in pregame warm-ups, and he makes eye contact with us; all is well. I'm thrilled to see Nate out on the field again, defending, positioning, directing teammates, and having fun. He's in his element. Looking back, I'm not quite sure how the game turned out—a win or loss. Hmm. No matter. It's a beautiful, sunny, blue-sky, warm autumn day, with trees overlooking the hillsides of the Hudson River lined with speckles of orange, red, and yellow. Not many leaves remaining but the breeze continued to delicately break them off of the tree branches while they gently fluttered down to the welcoming earth of the Hudson Valley. We're reveling in the moments!

Nate rushes back to take a shower, and forty-five minutes later we pick him up at Grant turnaround. The evening ends with catch-up conversations and family time over dinner at the Park Restaurant. Up next, our first football game at West Point, Army versus Temple in Michie Stadium.

Game day! The entryways to West Point are few and far in between, and when you throw Army Black Knight football into the mix, you get traffic. Lots of it!

Luckily, this visit has us staying at the West Point Motel on Main Street in Highland Falls. A quick and easy right turn out of the parking lot places us in the stop-and-go flow of cars. Another picture-perfect autumn day sees a lot of energetic, enthusiastic fans leisurely walking along Main Street and the West Point Highway toward the Thayer Gate entrance in front of Buffalo Soldier Field. It's an uphill hike from there to Michie Stadium for those brave enough to make the trek. For us, on the other hand, we're in possession of a parking pass to Lot F above Hollander Center, which serves as the home of the Army ice hockey team, and the Christl Arena, venue for the men's and women's basketball squads.

This is all familiar territory and brings back exciting memories from nine months earlier. Nate scheduled an overnight visit at West Point after receiving his congressional nomination letter from Representative Keith Rothfus, Twelfth District, Pennsylvania in December (2016). Nate pretty much had his mind made up about becoming an Army officer after spending a week at West Point during Summer Leader's Experience (SLE). SLE is a highly competitive program where approximately six thousand high school juniors compete for just one thousand slots annually. The program is focused on rising high school seniors interested in attending West Point. During the week-long training experience, participants live and train as cadets. Activities cover everything from reporting to the cadet in the red sash, field training, practice academics, marksmanship, and sleeping in the barracks.

After picking Nate up from his week at SLE, he let us know it was West Point or bust. So much so that he only checked one box on his congressional nomination application for the section that asks, "Which of the academies are you interested in attending? Please number according to your preference. You will be considered only for those academies for which you have indicated an interest, and in the order in which you have ranked them below."

Air Force __ Merchant Marine __ Naval __ Military __

Easy enough to figure out which box got marked with 1. Yep, military! And the others were left blank. Determined, persistent, resolute, and steadfast—this was the fabric of Nate's West Point journey.

* * *

It's Wednesday, January 18, 2017, and Cathy and I make our way into town to pick Nate and Sam up from school to make our trip to West Point for Nate's overnight visit on Thursday through noon on Friday. We pull into Somerset High School and sign the boys out of classes. Nate jumps into the car, runny nose and glassy eyes from a lingering cold, and shares some electrifying news with us.

"Hi, guess what?" he says. And then before we can answer, he hurriedly goes on to say he was paged to the main office to take a phone call from Representative Rothfus.

"Wow, that's amazing!" we say. "Why did he call?"

Nate says the congressman congratulated him on his nomination and next steps.

"Next steps?" I blurt out. "You got it, Nate! You got an appointment!"

"No, I don't think so," Nate answers.

We stop pressing him for more details. He's so stuffed up, and the cold symptoms seem to be taking their toll on him. Cathy brought a blanket and pillow along, and our plan is to let him rest. Hopefully, he'll feel well enough for the overnight stay.

Thursday morning finds Cathy, Nate, Sam, and me leaving our room at the Thayer Hotel to get IDs taken at the visitors' center. Not too busy at this hour. A few construction contractors in line ahead of us and we complete the task. And none too soon. We step outside and Nate runs to the nearest trash can and throws up. This cold is getting the better of him and he needs more rest. Poor guy. We talk him through calling the admissions office to let them know he's sick. To our surprise, they make arrangements for a day visit the next day, Friday, January 20. The admissions office informs Nate that there are several other candidates doing day visits and they'll match him up with a cadet for a half day. During the time he's away, parents can meet with the admissions officer and attend a briefing. Perfect! We have our list of questions ready. Things are falling into place, and a few minutes later, we tuck Nate into bed with a hot cup of tea and water by his side.

"Nate, we're going to visit the museum and eat lunch at Tony's Pizza," Cathy tells Nate as she feels his forehead and brushes back his curly hair. "Can we bring you anything back?"

"No, I'm fine. I'll just sleep," he answers.

"Okay, if you need anything, just give me a call," Cathy ends, with a final kiss on the top of his head.

The museum at West Point is such a magnificent place to visit. There are numerous exhibits and displays of large and small weapons, uniforms, and memorabilia of American soldiers from the seventeenth century to the present as well as military artifacts from around the world. Notable historic pieces include items from George Washington, Napoleon I, John Pershing, Dwight Eisenhower, George Patton, and Adolph Hitler. A stop at the museum is a must-see if you ever find yourself at West Point.

The pepperoni pizza and antipasto salad at Tony's were delicious, but we downplay our lunch outing with Nate. We get him some soup and crackers and hot tea from General Patton's Tavern (inside the Thayer Hotel) and are pleasantly surprised that he has an appetite; not much, but he's eating. The remainder of the day is spent mostly sequestered in the hotel room. Tomorrow is another day.

The admissions office is bustling with enthusiastic, anxious parents and cadet candidates, some already with appointments and others, like Nate, waiting to receive word. We're directed to a briefing room, and one by one, Nate and the other young men and women

are matched with West Point cadets dressed in their operational camouflage pattern (OCP) uniforms. And like a mirage, poof! They're
gone.

The admissions officer takes over. Introductions of himself
and two Firstie cadets. Informational packets are handed out, along
with black-speckled West Point coffee cups. And the sounds of shattered ceramic stoneware echoes within the room. "Oops," someone
exclaims. A replacement mug is quickly passed back to her, and the
morning overview continues on.

The Firsties speak with confidence and pride as they describe
the West Point experience. A day in the life of a cadet, campus activities, USMA traditions, cadet fitness, and other preparations for
becoming a commissioned US Army officer. The admissions officer
then asks if any of the parents would like to speak with him regarding their cadet's individual file assessment. Yes, we quickly raise our
hands and find ourselves second in line. Just like that, we're in. Cathy
and I introduce ourselves while Nate's file is being accessed. To our
surprise, the officer congratulates us on Nate receiving an appointment to the United States Military Academy at West Point. He's a bit
bewildered at our own perplexed faces and response.

"So it's official?" I ask in reply.

"Yes, sir," he politely responds with a big smile. Nate was
specified as the principal candidate for Pennsylvania's Twelfth
Congressional District, and he goes on to say, "Wow, an impressive
file. Did your congressman contact your son?" the admissions officer
further inquiries.

"Yes." Then we explain the sequence of events from two days
ago when we picked Nate up from school. Now it all makes perfect
sense. The telephone call from Rep. Rothfus was, in fact, a congratu-
latory call. I'm sure it caught Nate off guard. With that, the mystery
is solved. Crazy, our son has been accepted to one of the most distinguished institutions in the entire world and he doesn't even know it.
Now how do we share the wonderful, phenomenal news with Nate?

Sam comes to the rescue and says, "I'll tell Nate!" All three of us
are smiling ear to ear when Nate calls to let us know he just finished
with his cadet visit and tour.

"We'll meet you outside the admissions building," Cathy tells him.

Nate shares that he was escorted by a Plebe from Tennessee. A lot of fast-paced walking and intense schedules, he says.

We move to the walkway to the right of the admissions building, which leads to the cadet store, and tell Nate and Sam we want to take a picture of the two of them. Sam puts his arm around Nate's shoulder, both boys smiling, and says, "Nate, guess what?"

Nate answers with a quizzical, half-hearted smile, "What, Sam?"

"You're in! You got the appointment to West Point!" Sam proclaims.

Click. Cathy perfectly captures the moment. No more second-guessing, no more doubts or unknowns. This is the beginning of the momentous journey of Nate becoming a thread in the historic fabric of the Long Gray Line. But before all that happens, Friday evening is a time to celebrate and we do just that at MacArthur's Riverview Restaurant in the Thayer Hotel. We all order the seafood buffet and close out the day on full stomachs.

Saturday's plans include taking in two Army Black Knight games, women's basketball versus Navy, and men's hockey versus the Royal Military College of Canada. Two exciting games with the Black Knight women making a dramatic comeback only to lose in overtime. The men's hockey team saw a 5–3 victory at Tate Rink in front of a sellout crowd. Our first taste of Army athletics!

Word of Nate's good news is quickly finding its way to family and friends. And to our surprise, when we pull into our driveway at home on Sunday afternoon, we see the front porch decorated with black and gold balloons, streamers, and a huge banner also in black and gold, with the words Congratulations, Nate written on it. Who could have done this? Well, none other than Aunt Susie and Uncle Jim. Wow! They're so delighted and ecstatic for Nate. They've been so supportive all along and continue to play an integral role with Nate's West Point journey.

* * *

Now with those memories behind us, we once again find ourselves exiting our car in F lot, but instead of basketball and hockey, and winter and cold, it's fall football at USMA. Michie Stadium makes its debut with the Olsavskys. Hoodies, pumpkin spice, and tailgating. Are we anxious? You betcha!

Every college football fan should make it a point to see a game at West Point. A bucket-list item for sure. Arrive early to get to your seats to see the Army parachute team land midfield with the US flag and game ball. Yes, the Army parachute team jumps into the stadium, carrying the ball which is strapped to a cadet who jumps from a helicopter into Michie Stadium.

The helicopter flyby is timed near perfectly with the opening kickoff. There's no shortage of tradition for the Black Knights either. Army cadets do push-ups on the field and in the bleachers for every point the football team scores. But it's not seven push-ups or three for a field goal. Tradition dictates that cadets do push-ups for the total score each time new points are scored. Yikes! And with every touchdown, the West Point cannon crew celebrates with a volley of cannon fire over Lusk Reservoir.

Mel Kiper Jr., ESPN sports analyst, sums it up best: "There is nothing like being at Michie Stadium on the banks of the Hudson River with the leaves changing during the third weekend in October. The scenery is incredible. And how about the inspiration drawn from being at such a historic landmark? You see the statues of MacArthur, Patton, and Eisenhower. Then on game-day morning, you have the pleasure of witnessing the cadet parade. And how about when the cadets sing 'On Brave Old Army Team?' That is an unbelievable moment."

And this gorgeous fall October 17, 2017, Saturday does not disappoint. The Black Knights come from behind on the final seconds of regulation to tie the Temple Owls and then win in dramatic fashion with an overtime field goal, 31–28! Wow!

Cody, Stella, and Remi continue to entertain and provide a cornucopia of pics and backdrop subject matter for the next two volumes of Cadet Cody: Family Weekend at USMA-West Point and the buildup to Army versus Navy, December 9, 2017. Laughs galore and the themes keep us closely connected with Nate.

October soon ends; we change the clocks back one hour, and the Thanksgiving holiday is fast approaching. November delivers another first for our Plebe. A weekend visit to the United States Air Force Academy in Colorado Springs, Nate was tagged as one of the lucky ones to make the trip with the Club Soccer Team and go up against the AF Falcons squad. The Black Knights have a full schedule of games planned to include their first challenge to hold on to the CIC Trophy. Nate's soccer game is on Friday, November 3, and after that, relax and enjoy time with his AF Academy hosts and the opportunity to take in some of the unique sights.

Before that, however, Thursday presents a fine spectacle of West Point cadet activity as they make their way in bus after bus to Stewart International Airport located in Orange County, New York, in the southern Hudson Valley, west of Newburgh, and southwest of Poughkeepsie. Nate's first flight on a military transport plane, with the exception of him and Sam, taxiing around in the C-130 Tactical Transport Aircraft at Pittsburgh's 911th Airlift Wing for Sam's Pilot for a Day program. To think that was only a few months ago.

Nate sends us a wonderful picture of him standing on the stadium turf, dressed in his warm-up sweatshirt, with a magnificent backdrop of colors—yellow, gold, orange, and red hues—as the sun fades away with him framed in among the Colorado Rocky Mountains. Simply amazing! Oh, and Army won the club soccer game. I wouldn't want to pass up an opportunity to mention that fact. Up next, an inter-academy bonfire in anticipation of tomorrow's football game.

Saturday, November 4, does not disappoint. For the Army Black Knights, that is. Army's quarterback rushed for a career-high 265 yards and Army's defense ended Air Force's 306-game scoring streak in a 21–0 win.

With the return from Colorado Springs, club soccer season closes out without fanfare, and on the academic front, Nate lets us know that he's excelling. First semester at USMA and all is well. So far so good!

"Guess what came in the mail today?" Cathy enthusiastically blurts out while, at the same time, waving a rectangular-shaped envelope addressed from WPAOG, the West Point Association of Graduates.

"Army-Navy tickets! Yay," she continues on. The game is just a little over a month away, December 9, at Lincoln Financial Field in Philadelphia. Her logistics expertise is in full swing now but a few questions to answer. Where to stay? When do we leave? Are we going to tailgate? Will we be able to meet up with Nate? Our first Army-Nave football game! Last year, with Nate having a congressional nomination but no appointment, we watched the game from the comforts of our living room. And in a turnover-filled 21-17 loss, Navy's fourteen-game winning streak over Army, a series record, came to an end. Pure excitement watching from home and now we'll be part of what is considered to be the most singular bucket-list game in all sports.

Before Thanksgiving comes around, however, this November throws an extra piece of drama our way. A friend of mine convinced me to pursue an open director seat on the Somerset Area School District School Board. It was too late to get my name put on the ballots, so I had to push ahead with a write-in campaign. My baptism by fire with local politics. Too funny!

Tuesday, election day, November 7, arrives, and Cathy and I find ourselves at our voting district, handing out flyers colored in orange and black (the school colors) written with Elect Joe Olsavsky, Write-In Candidate, Somerset Area School Board.

A few weeks later and as fate (or luck) would have it, I receive a letter from the board of election with notice that I have become one of two new school board director members. Pretty cool stuff!

We're coming down the final stretch of the year and it's quite astounding to reflect on what we've experienced. Our first family pet with Cody, Sam's surgery, Nate's appointment to West Point, Hillary and Jacob becoming new homeowners, another car, and now me becoming a member of the local school board.

The next three weeks fly by and Thanksgiving is upon us. We avert making a trip to West Point to pick Nate up or putting him on the Western Pennsylvania West Point Parents' Club bus for drop-off in Pittsburgh. How? Well, Nate is catching a ride back to Somerset with a family driving through our area, and we meet for dinner at the Pine Grill Restaurant with them and our cadet boys.

The conversation quickly moves from our menu selections, on to how the boys are coping with the demands of Plebe year, and then to discussion of none other than the game. Yes, the Army-Navy game! We share Thanksgiving dinner plans for tomorrow and are strategizing on getting together in a few weeks on the Friday evening before the game. And just like that, turkey day is upon us.

"Good morning. Happy Thanksgiving," Cathy softly whispers as her iPhone alarm sounds off. It is 5:00 AM and we gingerly make our way downstairs to the kitchen. This has been our holiday routine for many, many years now. And unlike previous years, it seems like we have an extra adrenaline kick with Nate home. For all that, however, nothing takes the place of the programmable coffee maker. A fresh, hot pot of coffee greets us as we turn on the lights in the kitchen. Yeah, the first cup of coffee helps our sequenced preparation for a traditional Thanksgiving dinner: roast turkey, stuffing, mashed potatoes, gravy, green bean casserole, buttered corn, sweet potato casserole, dinner rolls, cranberry sauce, pumpkin and apple pie with whipped cream, and a fruit, cheese, and vegetable tray to nibble on as appetizers. The turkey is in the oven!

Another part of the tradition includes playing Christmas music as we work in sync between the kitchen and dining room. Now wait for it; we go old-school and play vinyl record albums on a vintage Scott-model stereo receiver and turntable. The crackling, popping, and bump sound when the needle is moved over the album can't be beat. Bing Crosby's "White Christmas," Elvis Presley's "Blue Christmas," Andy Williams' "It's the Most Wonderful Time of the Year," and Eartha Kitt's "Santa Baby" are just a few throwback classics that softly play in the background.

Cody wakes up, and his tiny nose is in overdrive with the luscious smells permeating the house. And speaking of an aromatic wake-up call, the scents lure our sleepy boys out of their beds and into the kitchen where they indulge themselves with a slice of pie.

Nate and I go to 9:00 AM Mass at St. Peter's and then make a stop to pick up newspapers containing all the Black Friday sales flyers. These are must-have items for later this evening, particularly when Cathy, Hillary, and Cathy's siblings plot out their early Friday-morning game plan to shop. We proceed to Sheetz, a food and fuel convenience store where we luckily find the newspapers. Mission accomplished!

Hillary and Jacob, along with Stella and Remi, arrive at the house not long after Pap shows up. Sam finished making his home-made cranberry sauce earlier, and it's perfectly chilled. Now the only thing left to do is give thanks, sit back, and enjoy Thanksgiving dinner—delicious food and enjoyable conversation, all in plentiful supply. Ours is the complete opposite of *A Charlie Brown Thanksgiving*: "I can't cook a Thanksgiving dinner. All I can make is cold cereal and maybe toast" (Charlie Brown). Year after year, Cathy outdoes herself, and this year is no exception. Are we thankful? Sam is healthy, Cody is an absolute joy, Nate is doing well at West Point, and Hillary is on her way—a young, successful, happily married homeowner. Are we thankful and grateful enough? Absolutely. Life is definitely good.

Black Friday and Thanksgiving and now one- and two-day old memories. Now Saturday's heavy chill but dry weather gives us an opportunity to get outdoors for a spell. Hillary takes the lead and barks out orders to Sam and Nate, telling them that Mom and Dad want to do a family hike at Laurel Hill State Park. Hiking boots, hats, gloves, and a few snacks, along with bottled water, find their way into our backpacks. And Hillary and Sam, our resident family photographers, bring their Nikon D3400 and Canon EOS80D DSLR (digital single-lens reflex) cameras along for what I'm sure will be numerous photo-op moments. Pictures aside, it'll be nice just spending time together. Cathy and I know these occasions, where all five of us are out and about together for any length of time, are passing swiftly by. Our wonderful, gifted, and blessed kids are growing up.

We drive along Trent Road to enter the park and decide to hike Pumphouse Trail in the Hemlock Trail Natural Area of Laurel Hill. Nowhere to be today and nothing to rush us. We find our rhythm in a leisurely pace along Pumphouse Trail and take a break at Jones Mill

Run Dam. And the cameras are in full motion. The water is crystal clear, and to our surprise, we see a few trout at the front of the dam. Neat stuff! And these pictures find their way into *The Adventure of Cadet Cody*. I more clearly see what my mom and dad saw with us *ten little Indians*: me, my five sisters, and four brothers. In their eyes, we were considered priceless gems, each in our own unique way. These emotions resonate with Cathy and me as we secretly, simply watch Sam, Nate, and Hillary making small talk as they move through the oaks, hemlocks, maple, cherry, and poplar trees, throwing sticks, observing the waterfall, and snapping pictures.

Sibling relationships are authentic. Hillary, Nate, and Sam, while being separated by time and distance, and now in the midst of independent lives, genuinely show their love for one another. Cathy and I take it all in, the pure, incalculable reward of being parents. Words can't describe these feelings. And the three of them have so much more ahead of them. "The sibling relationship is life's longest lasting relationship, longer for most of us by a quarter of a century, than our ties to our parents," wrote Stephen Bank and Michael Kahn in the *Sibling Bond*. "It lasts longer than our relationship with our children, certainly longer than with a spouse and, with the exception of a few lucky men and women, longer than with a best friend."

The moment has arrived! Game day! Today, we'll be part of the historic 118th meeting between Army and Navy. It's a game everyone feels good watching as these are the cadets and midshipmen, soon-to-be Army second lieutenants and Navy ensigns, who will defend our country after graduation.

Rivalry games often mean teams breaking out specialty uniforms for the occasion, and this year is no exception for the Black Knights. The 2017 Army-Navy specialty uniform tells the story of the soldiers of the Tenth Mountain Division and their birth in the winter warfare of World War II. The Tenth Mountain Division is a light infantry division based at Fort Drum, New York. It is the only one of its size in the US military to receive intense specialized training for fighting in mountainous and arctic conditions.

The uniforms, called Climb to Glory, honor the alpine soldiers who fought the Nazis in the Alps of Italy. The white helmets, white pants, and white jerseys mimic the camouflage the soldiers wore to blend in with the snow. I don't think this could have been planned any better to offer special tribute to the Climb to Glory uniforms. The forecast for today in Philadelphia—snow.

Transportation is arranged for the boys to Lincoln Financial Field this morning for the cadet accountability and pregame lineup. Before drop-off, however, the boys are treated to coffee and ham, sausage, bacon, egg and cheese breakfast sandwiches at a favorite breakfast stop. No complaints from our cadets.

And to no one's surprise, Cathy's extraordinary planning skills find us with a parking pass in M-Lot and tickets to a tailgate party sponsored by the West Point Parents' Club of New Jersey. The parking lot is abuzz with activity—vendors selling T-shirts, hats, banners, and scarves; cornhole boards, along with charcoal and propane grills, abound; and the smell of hot dogs, hamburgers, beer, and some interesting hard liquor bar setups. Army-West Point memorabilia—flags, coasters, cups, towels—are everywhere. This is the year of the *repeat*. Or at least we hope. The Navy ice sculpture fountain still sticks with me to this day. The shot of fireball cinnamon whiskey went a long way in the friendly conversation with my Navy host, ending with each of us wishing both Army and Navy well today.

It's 11:00 AM and the lines at the gates are building in anticipation of march on tentatively planned for noon. Before the kickoff of every Army-Navy game, the cadets of the US Military Academy at West Point and the midshipmen of the US Naval Academy take the field. No, not just the football teams playing that day; the entire student body, nearly nine thousand strong, march on the field in the way only disciplined, drilled, and trained US troops can. Together they stand. Determined, committed, and unstoppable in their charge to defend those in the stands today and everywhere else throughout America and the world. We are ready. We will march on! What does this mean? One needs to look no further than a quote from General Douglas MacArthur, a West Point graduate and renowned military leader. MacArthur's quote, which is immortalized in West Point lore and chiseled in granite between Michie Stadium and Hollander Athletic Center, reads, "Upon the fields of friendly strife are sown the seeds that on other days, on other fields, will bear the fruits of victory."

Today, however, we're here to watch our cadet Nate march on to the field for the very first time dressed in his West Point long overcoat. This is part of the uniform that West Point cadets wear to each Army-Navy football game every year. We pass through the initial entrance to the stadium gates and are surrounded by pageantry of all sorts. Uniform display booths, bands playing, vendors, Humvee and weapon displays, and a pull-up competition. Crazy! But all good spirited.

The temperature continues to drop, and the sky has turned from the flat gray color of the West Point cadet uniforms to now being speckled with those individual unique frozen-water crystals. Yep, it's snowing! Big snowflakes, heavy wet flakes are thinly and exquisitely blanketing the stadium seats as we make our way through the south gate and proceed toward the southeast section of the stadium—section M13, rows 15 and 16 in the end zone. Now seated, we begin to take in even more of the Army-Navy rivalry grandeur and fanfare.

To be honest, before Nate received his appointment, I never had an interest in the game. The Army-Navy rivalry isn't for everyone, and my only recollection goes way back to grade school when my dad would turn on the television and follow the game—this game and Notre Dame football. Funny thing, he didn't much care for Pitt or Penn State, but Notre Dame was his team. Nate didn't have the opportunity to know his grandfather; he passed away in the fall before Nate was born. But they share a common bond. Or should I say several bonds? Both soldiers in the United States Army. Nate and his grandfather share the same middle name: Joseph. And what is Nate's closest tie with his grandfather? They were born on the same day. Seventy-six years apart.

I can only imagine how proud and honored my dad would be if he was alive. It would have been amazing to walk the grounds of West Point with him, as well as the West Point Museum and Cemetery, Eisenhower Hall, and Constitution Island, and to look at the statues of MacArthur, Patton, and Grant, along with Battle Monument,

Buckner Monument, Cadet Monument, and Custer and Eisenhower Monuments. And a scenic overview visit to Trophy Point and a stop at the Thomas Jefferson Hall—US Military Academy Library and Learning Center. I'm absolutely certain Dad would have loved the rolling hills, building architecture, and other sights that only the Hudson Valley at USMA offers. And like me, he would have been wearing West Point attire—a hat, jacket, shirt, proudly broadcasting to the world, "I have a grandson in the Army, he's at West Point."

And as the Lincoln Financial Field end zones disappeared under a coating of snow, the rest of the gridiron is now revealing the footsteps of the Corps of Cadets. The First, Second, Third, and Fourth Regiments and their commanding officers are announced over the stadium speakers, along with the company commanders, cadet first captain, cadet first sergeants, and others. Simply an incredible experience! Cathy and I think to ourselves, *Will Nate one day earn one of these key leadership roles and have his name announced in front of tens of thousands of people and a national TV audience?* Only time will tell. Navy's Brigades of Midshipmen, in much the same way, make their way onto the field. Game time is fast approaching, and now this East Coast weather is setting the stage for the football game to be played in a snow globe. Interestingly, the only site west of the Mississippi River to host the Army-Navy game was the Rose Bowl in 1983. No snow at that game!

Cathy directs us farther down on the bleachers in the mezzanine level—better photo optics looking over the field. A few pics later, we hear someone calling, "Cathy, Cathy," trying to get her attention. What do you know? It's one of her girlfriends from Somerset, here with her family to watch the game. Such a small world. After a few minutes of friendly conversation in the falling, wet snow and asking about Nate, we make our way back to our seats. Everyone is gearing up already in an attempt to stay warm and dry. We shall see.

Cathy's phone is ringing, and it's Nate! "Hi, Mom," he says. "Can I meet up with you guys now?" Nate asks. "I have time before kickoff, so I can come over."

"We'll meet you at the concession stand in M13," Cathy tells him. Perfect! This is an extra bonus for us. We're like kids at Christmas as we rush out of our seats and walk toward the concession area. In short order, we're all together! Nate looks great, looking so handsome dressed in his uniform with the long gray overcoat. More often than not, this is the vision most people have of the young men and women who make up the Long Gray Line.

We buy Nate a steak and cheese hoagie, French fries, and a Coke. Amazing how quickly that boy can devour food! Our friends from Somerset come over to chat and see how he's doing. I think they're just as excited as us to see Nate. How can you not be caught up in all the excitement? Something words cannot describe. And as quick as Nate arrived, he has to make his way back.

The snow has put a damper on the Army and Navy parachute teams, and the pregame jumps are cancelled and also the Army helicopter and Navy jet flyover. Yes, snow in Philly has gotten the better of these two magnificent pregame events. Darn! We'll have to wait until next year. But all is not lost. The prisoner exchange is underway! That's right, the game begins with a prisoner exchange. During the fall semester, West Point and the Naval Academy swap some of their students, along with the US Air Force and Coast Guard academies so that each side engenders respect and a better understanding of what the respective branches do. During the Army-Navy game, those who have been experiencing the *culture* of the other side ceremonially cross the field for an ad hoc release to their fellow cadets and midshipmen. Seven members each from corps and brigades meet up at midfield. The cadets in gray display REPEAT written out in yellow tape on the back of their overcoats; and the seven Navy exchange prisoners advertise REVENGE, crisply spelled in yellow tape as well. These fourteen young men and women crazily dash to their respective sides of the field. And why the madness and delirium? Why? Because the Commander in Chief's Trophy (CIC), one of college football's unique rivalry trophies, is at stake. That and bragging rights, of course!

The CIC Trophy is the three-way prize for the service academy that comes out on top—one of the sport's most prestigious. The trophy gets awarded to either the Army, Navy, or Air Force academy that wins the triple-threat match between the schools. If the competition is tied, the previous year's winner retains it. This year is a remarkably different story. After Army's shutout of Air Force (21–0) and Navy's win over the Falcons, Army-Navy is an all-out, legit trophy game. Yes, the Commander in Chief's Trophy is on the line!

Kickoff time. Here we go! Instead of rain, we have snow and wind. A great start nonetheless. Because on Army's opening drive, in uniforms matching the snow on the field, they crunch and grind their way to a touchdown. Army finds the end zone. Army 7, Navy 0. Things are off to a great start. Now Navy, with only 55 seconds left in the first quarter, elects to settle for a field goal instead of making a go for it on fourth and 2.

Early into the start of the second quarter, the quarterback turned slotback rips off a 68-yard touchdown run. Navy 10, Army 7. Things are getting interesting and everything about America's Game is living up to expectations. And we get a snow game, with it expected to keep coming down the entire game. Halftime finds us cold and wet. The blankets, hand warmers, seat pads, and extra hats certainly help, but this snow is unforgiving. Surprisingly, the concession stands aren't too jam-packed. The same cannot be said for the restrooms. Total insanity! And not in the sense of everyone needing to empty their bladders. Nope. The restrooms are heated, and hot air is blowing from the ceiling vents. Crowded is an understatement. We grab a bite to eat and make our way in and out of the restrooms to warm up. My shoulders and neck are so tense from trying to stay warm, shaking off the heavy wet snow in between shivers.

Navy fans are beginning to feel like revenge may be within reach as they go up 13–7 less than halfway through the third quarter. And to start the fourth quarter, Army drives into the red zone and stalls on a third and long. A missed field goal by Army's kicker begins the fourth quarter. Like the dismal weather, we are feeling much the same, along with our fellow Army brethren.

Cathy and Sam have reached their limit. Freezing, wet, tired, and just maxed out from a roller-coaster type of day, they throw in the towel and tap out. "We're going to the car to warm up," Cathy tells us. "We'll listen to the rest of the game on the radio." I give her a kiss and we say our goodbyes as the enormous snowflakes show no sign of stopping.

But things begin to turn from bad to better after a Navy three and out drive. Army's elusive and outstanding rusher, with the moniker of quarterback, takes it from Army's 35-yard line on a seven-and-a-half-minute drive on multiple runs and finds his way into Navy's end zone! At 5:10 of the fourth quarter, Army goes up 14–13! The entire stadium is on their feet. And like a scripted, made-for-TV drama, Navy makes a final drive to get within field goal range; and with three seconds showing on the clock, it comes down to this. All or nothing. Navy's placekicker sets up for 48-yard field goal attempt for the win.

And as time expires with Navy having the distance, the ball goes left giving Army a 14–13 victory before a crowd of 68,625 and possession of the Commander in Chief's Trophy for the first time since 1996. Army beats Navy for the second year in a row, this time on a missed kick at the buzzer. No matter what the outcome of the annual Army-Navy game, the day always ends the same way—honoring the fallen. The players sing both team's alma maters. The winners will join the losing team, facing the losing side's fans. Then the two groups will do the same for the winning team. It's a simple act of respectful sportsmanship that reminds everyone that today was a game played *upon the fields of friendly strife*. This year, Army sings second!

With everyone being borderline hypothermic, we begin our march out of Lincoln Financial Stadium. Army fans elated, Navy fans replaying that kick over and over and over again in their minds. We find Nate outside the stadium and walk to the car. How would we rate our first Army-Navy game experience? Magnificent!

The buildup to Christmas is underway. Nate is getting anxious to finish out his first semester and the TEE (term-end exam) schedules have been finalized. It looks like we'll get our cadet back home on December 21. Like so many traditions and other firsts Nate has experienced already, up next is the annual Corps of Cadets Christmas Dinner slotted for Thursday, December 14. Every cadet is assigned to a specific dining table in Washington Hall, and tradition dictates that the Plebes decorate their respective table and also provide gifts for everyone seated there. Nate is already ahead of the game. Over Thanksgiving break, Cathy took him on a Christmas shopping spree to pick up an assortment of decorations—a lighted tree, chair covers, Christmas tablecloth, candy canes, snowmen, lights, stockings, and a small gift for all the older classmen, such as Matchbox racing cars and plastic Army men. However, the pièce de résistance is the post-dinner ceremonial walk outside of Washington Hall to the Plain and surrounding area. Why? Every year, in addition to decorating the tables in festive fashion, the Plebes get cigars for the upperclassman at the table, and after dinner, the entire Corps of Cadets goes outside to smoke their cigars, celebrate Christmas, and enjoy some holiday fireworks!

Nate is sending us some pictures of the pre-decorating work taking place in Washington Hall—Plebes dressed in their ACUs, all smiles, laughing, and decorations of all sorts, such as flashing lights, toys, balloon, figurines, trees, holiday plates, and cups, etc.

Cathy, showing a huge smile, updates me, "Look at this. Nate's table is on the West Point Instagram page! That's his table, right?" she asks me.

"Wow, yep, that's it for sure!" I say. How cool is that! Honestly, for Nate and his fellow Plebes, it seems like everything is a *first of firsts*. The corps is dressed in their full-dress gray uniforms to celebrate Christmas and showing their pent-up anticipation of their upcoming TEEs and Christmas break. Nate sends us pictures of him smoking a cigar near the Plain, and with that, another volume of Cadet Cody comes to life: "Merry Christmas from the Corps of Cadets!" Two memorable callouts in the story included, "But Cadet Cody and Cadet Olsavsky's Christmas spirit begin to grow, and along with the Grinch, they begin to sing and their hearts are aglow."

And Cadet Cody replies, with a picture of Nate in his white Beat Navy T-shirt, "From me and Cadet Olsavsky, Merry Christmas, Navy, and Happy New Year!"

All is well with the ongoing pleasant and memorable events for our cadet. Such was not the case in the early year of the academy during the Christmas week of 1826. Over the Christmas holiday, several cadets smuggled a large quantity of whiskey into West Point to make some homemade eggnog and take a break from the grueling regimen of cadet life. The Eggnog Riot, as it became known, was the resultant aftermath that took place on December 24–25, 1826. The riot involved more than one-third of the cadets by the time it ended on Christmas morning. A subsequent investigation by officials resulted in the court-martialing of twenty cadets. One of the most notable participants, although not court-martialed, was future Confederate States President Jefferson Davis.

Nate's period of confinement comes to an end as his week of TEEs wrap up—check the box on MA153 differential equations, IT105 intro to programming, EN101 English 1, CH151 advanced general chemistry, and LF371 advanced intermediate French. Now our focus is on getting Nate back home for the Christmas and New Year holidays. And our good deed from several months ago, Labor Day weekend, is returned in kind by a West Point Parents' Club mom. She offers to pick up her two daughters and Nate on Thursday afternoon, December 21. We are saved a trip to West Point and make plans to meet up off Interstate 80 at Exit 161, US220S, to Bellefonte and State College, Pennsylvania.

At 10:30 PM that evening, as we wait in a parking lot, we see a van approaching our way. Yep, it's them! Cathy presents a Christmas basket as a small token of our thanks, and after a few minutes of small talk, holiday well-wishes, and parting hugs, everyone is on their way—homeward bound. A much-needed and overdue schedule of sleeping in, perfectly planned meals, accompanied by overeating, catch-up time with family and friends, and endless breaks of boredom for our children and the rest of the Corps of Cadets. Our kids are back in the comfort of their homes. Merry Christmas and Happy New Year!

CHAPTER 6

Plebe Parent Weekend and Staying Strong

A TEXT MESSAGE appears on our phones. It's from Nate. <Cathy and Joe. 4:00 PM.> "I'm back in my room. We made it back okay. Thanks for a wonderful break. I miss you guys already. Love you." The holidays just flew by; it seems like we just picked Nate up. I guess that is a sign we had a wonderful time.

And speaking of time, our membership in the West Point Parents' Club of Western Pennsylvania saves us hours on the road. We bought Nate a ticket for the coach bus ride back to West Point for the cadets in Western Pennsylvania and surrounding areas. Such a huge convenience!

For now, though, January finds us deep in the throes of winter. Here at home, Sam continues to work part-time at Hidden Valley Ski Resort, putting in many hours at the rental shop, and Nate is confined to the isolation of West Point, along with the persistent gray atmosphere and the blandness of the gray winter days. From January through March, everything at West Point is gray—uniforms, buildings, the Hudson Valley mountains, and the weather. Nevertheless, the first few days after winter leave finds the cadets in Winter Reorganization Week. The cadets get new rooms, some choose new roommates, new jobs for upperclassmen, and homework assignments. Plebe duties, room management, and personal military

123

inspections (SAMI)—Saturday morning (AM) inspections continue just like the first semester.

Our agreed-upon check-ins with Nate keep us up-to-date with all the latest happenings at West Point. Like clockwork, he calls us Sunday afternoon, once per week. He knows that we are available anytime. This touchpoint becomes another part of his fine-tuned structured routine. Moreover, one less thing to worry about for now is company athletics. There is a short respite from company sports until the Corps of Cadets return from spring break in mid-March. No complaints from him with having a little extra time. We, on the other hand, do have a complaint with Nate holding back information. As you can imagine, we have been so engrossed with news and updates of any kind. This includes clothing. The elusive cadet parka tops the list. All we have seen are pics of Nate wearing his Army ACU ECWCS (extended cold-weather clothing system) fleece. Then he sends it—a picture of the dark black jacket, the cadet parka, with a USMA 21 patch over the left breast and made with thirty-two ounces of heat-blanketing wool! *Sweet Baby Jesus!* A phrase Nate likes to use as he blazons in his excitement. Volume 8 of Cadet Cody finds an easy callout.

What we're not hearing about though is boxing. The entire Corps of Cadets are required to take boxing, including female cadets who entered the ring for the first time in 2016. Boxing is part of the physical curriculum at West Point and teaches hand-to-hand combative skills with the goal of improving the Warrior Ethos, confidence, and lethality. Cadets are evaluated in one-on-one, full-contact graded bouts consisting of two rounds that last a minute each. Boxing and combative at West Point are the only mandatory activity that pits one cadet against another in full-body contact. The end game? Fear management. Through boxing and combative, cadets learn to manage fear and perform physically despite the presence of enormous strength, a key quality necessary for combat leadership. The end game for Cathy? Well, this will not come until the second half of the semester. Nate assured Cathy that he would not say a single word about boxing—bloody noses, black eyes, broken ribs, concussions, or the likes—until he finishes the combative program. May is so very far away. Thank goodness.

January's cold and piercing days give way to February, and we are soon rewarded with President's Day weekend. A three-day respite, February 17–19, but better yet, a getaway to see Nate. No complaints from Sam either. He has been going gangbusters working at Hidden Valley; a few days off from work is bringing smiles to his face. Cathy makes reservations for the Holiday Inn Express in Fort Montgomery, along with May's Country Kennel; we take Cody to the kennel first thing Friday morning. Poor little guy. Cody gets anxious and a little separation anxiety when we leave. But the reunions with our lil' buddy are the best! Words cannot explain our joy when Cody comes running out from the back room at the kennel, his little tail wagging like a rattlesnake. Always a nice pick-me-up after leaving Nate knowing we have a tiny bundle of love waiting for us upon our return.

Saturday morning breakfast is relaxing, and we lay out plans for the day. A trip to Woodbury Commons Premium Outlets, a short thirty-minute drive away. Woodbury Commons is a major attraction for all kinds of visitors, West Pointers included, due to its proximity to New York City. The second part of our plan includes dinner reservations at Bear Mountain Inn.

Parking at the outlets is insane to say the least. No surprise with it being a holiday weekend. Several loops in and out of a few lots and, voilà, an open space! With jackets and hats in tow, a cold overcast day with snow in the forecast, we find our way to the visitor's center for a map to outline what stores to visit. Shopping can wait, though, for good reason. Planted directly in front of us are three electric full-body recliner chairs. One dollar gets three-minutes of an awesome massage. Sam, Nate, and I feed the chairs crisp one-dollar bills, and the contour and rolling vibration of the chairs begin to relax our muscles by stimulating blood flow. My lower back pain is quickly being erased. I'm tempted to sit here with $20 and have Cathy and the boys meet back up with me in an hour. Oh well, not to be. We feed three more $1 bills into the chairs and we readily see Cathy's amusement with her boys turning into "Let's get the show on the road." It's time to shop! Moreover, yes, as much as I hate to admit it, I enjoy the jaunt throughout the various outlet shops. PS: not as much as the West Point gift shops though.

At 5:30 PM, dinner reservations at Restaurant 1915 and Blue Roof Tapas Bar at Bear Mountain Inn arrives quickly. A group of eight round out our party—Cathy, Sam, and I, along with Nate and four of his friends. As Plebes, they are required to be in their dress gray uniforms. What an honor being surrounded by five handsome, incredible young men. Make that six! Our son Sam has blossomed into an extremely handsome, marvelous, wonderful young man in his own right. I think he takes all our attention with a grain of salt. On one hand, he hates being smothered by Cathy and me, being the center of attention. On the other hand, secretly, sometimes he shows his emotions. "Hey, this isn't too bad!" All part of life's many new beginnings that each and every one of us experience throughout the course of our lives.

Snow is showing on the weather app, due to arrive in the next two to three hours. However, that doesn't deter us as we pick up the boys in Grant turnaround. Driving five uniformed West Point cadets, taking them to dinner, who can complain? Easy enough to see how these cool, confident, fine-looking future Army officer specimens become show pieces for us.

As we enter the lobby of Bear Mountain Inn, a young lady dressed in Army athletic gear asks, "Hi, are you all heading back to West Point?"

"No," Cathy tells her and then goes on to invite her to dinner. "Would you like to join us for dinner?" Cathy inquires. "We can give you a ride back afterward if you'd like."

"No, thank you," the young woman replies as she starts looking at her cell phone again.

No shortage of kindness from Cathy. These moments always make me smile and I commit these occasions to memory. Such a joy to see simple acts of generosity and expressions of caring from Cathy, it warms the heart.

Once we're seated, menus in hand, Cathy tells Nate and his friends, "Don't be shy and help yourself to anything you see on the menu." Sam already has his mind made up. He has been thinking about having a medium-rare steak all day long, accompanied by a baked potato and butter. Sam is definitely a "meat and potatoes" kind of guy.

Conversation easily begins to flow among the boys, and Cathy and I balance any lull in the banter. We can't help ourselves and pry a bit with our questions. We're anxious to know where each cadet is from and learn a little about them. Uncommonly, they are all from the south. They briefly touch upon their West Point journeys, but mostly fill the table discussion with various happenings about PT, classes, instructors, and other cadets. Laughter is not in short supply, and they each ping Sam, asking him how school is going, what he likes about his part-time job, and what is in store with his future plans. Sam is all about rockets, faraway galaxies, life on other planets, NASA, and SpaceX. Aerospace engineering has come up on several occasions, so time will tell. Hillary, Nate, and Sam—our three fantastic children. Yes, we're proud parents! And we're glad to extend some parental warmth to Nate's friends this evening even if it only amounts to a few hours away from USMA. The boys leave no doubt about their appetites as we view clean plates and menu gazing at the dessert list.

Once again, we let the boys know that they can help themselves and egg them on. "Order away. Don't be shy," we tell them. It's easy to read between the lines that they miss their siblings, family and friends, and, yes, their pets. If but for a few hours, we're delighted to host our newfound cadet guests and listen to their stories—their ups and downs, triumphs, a few struggles, and a brief entry into their family background, each unique but so very similar to our own story.

Remember that weather forecast I mentioned earlier? Yes, it has arrived. We glanced outside through the huge glass windows in the restaurant periodically as the massive, feathery, iridescent white snowflakes begin to fall. Now in less than two hours, we are looking at several inches blanketing all the cars in the parking lot. A vibrant, picturesque, immaculate snow globe scene captivates us as we slowly make our way out into the awaiting storm.

"I'll have you guys wait here and I'll bring the car around," I tell the group. No need for everyone to get their feet soaking wet by trampling through the steeling snow. They gladly take me up on my offer. I cautiously navigate the unplowed 9W highway as we return back to West Point. The snow is falling as if each flake is a piece of fine metal and the ground, a magnet. Our southern cadet guests aren't going to let an opportunity like this pass by without some boyish mischief. No sooner than jumping over Sam and Nate to exit the car at Grant turnaround, the snowballs begin to fly. Oh yes, perfect snowball snow. I glance at the guard on duty inside the guardhouse and see a chuckle. Yes, boys will be boys.

We have the swimming pool to ourselves at the hotel, at least Sam and Nate do. Cathy and I watch from the comfort of our table and chairs as they enjoy the solitude of the water. They're making the most of every minute, a genuine brotherly rapport and enjoyable bro time.

Sunday morning allows a few extra hours of sleep for all of us. So nice. Today's plans—peruse the Palisades Center in West Nyack, New York, and take in dinner and a movie. Surprisingly, after last night's winter onslaught, the roads are now dry and clear. Blue sky and sunshine, along with temps approaching 40°F, are a welcome sight. What a difference from the whiteout yesterday evening.

"Can you believe the layout of the Palisades Mall?" Cathy asks us. "Four levels, the ice rink and bowling alley. Wow!" she continues.

"Yeah, that was pretty cool," Sam says.

"Did you like the movie, Nate?" I ask.

"It was really good. I've been wanting to see it," he replies.

After dinner, we decided to see *The 15:17 to Paris*, featuring Anthony Sadler, former Oregon Nationals Guardsman Alek Skarlatos, and Air Force veteran Spencer Stone. The movie depicts the three friends' vacation in Europe who ultimately help thwart a terrorist attack on a Paris-bound train. Salty, buttered popcorn topped off a great movie and a great day with our sons. Another item checked off our President's Day weekend list. And just like that, we now come to the last item on our checklist—hugs, kisses, goodbyes, and a final "love you, be safe" to Nate. Saying goodbye is never easy, and sadly, at many points in our lives, goodbyes are an inevitable part of life. This ending will be relatively brief, however, because our next time to say hello and meet up with Nate again will be Plebe Parent Weekend, scheduled for March 8–11, 2018. Perfect!

M*A*S*H, the 1970s dramatic comedy TV series that saw members of the 4077th Mobile Army Surgical Hospital care for the injured during the Korean War and use humor to escape from the horrors and depression of the situation, has always been a family favorite. Like so many others, my adolescent years were spent glued in front of the TV to watch the newest episode. The adult humor and underlying serious raw human themes are much more appreciated these days but, nonetheless, provided me with years of weekly laughter. Years gone by, yes, and now moments to share with two new fans—Sam and Nate. Sam gets such a kick out of the characters Hawkeye, BJ, Hot Lips, Klinger, Radar, and more, but particularly Major Frank Burns, nicknamed Ferret Face. One of my favorite episodes is from 1976 called "The Interview." The war correspondent interviewing Hawkeye asks him, "Is there anything from home that you brought over with you to set up for yourself? Creature comforts?"

Hawkeye responds, "I brought… I brought a book over."

Interviewer: "What book?"

Hawkeye: "The dictionary. I figure it's got all the books in it. I like to read the dictionary." Thank goodness for MeTV, America's place to watch a variety of classic television programs.

On February 27, 2018, Nate joins a packed house of 150 other cadets to listen to and meet Alan Alda, a.k.a. Captain Hawkeye Pierce. The *M*A*S*H* actor and author delivered a talk organized by the Modern War Institute to discuss the importance of communication while speaking to humans' innate ability to read others' minds. Alda joked with the audience, saying they might be wondering why West Point invited him. "They've taught you everything you need to know to be an officer. Now I'll teach you how to act like one." He tells them Hawkeye Pierce has come a long, long way!

Once again, our enthusiasm and anticipation come to fruition. An early morning drop-off at the kennel for Cody and by Thursday evening, March 7, passing through the Thayer Gates, we pull up to the Historic Thayer Hotel at West Point. Coming full circle, the last time here in January, was when Nate received his appointment.

Yeah, this place instantly triggers a flood of fantastic memories. Even the small things have that effect. You don't have to look any further than the refrigerator magnet in our kitchen. A small rectangular yellow-brown magnet with the words *My kid is having a BEAST of a summer. Class of 2021*. Every so often, I'll take a wistful look at those words and my thoughts serenely travel back to R-Day. What a wild ride it has been, and it continues on.

Now tired and drained, and after a few leg and arm stretches, it feels comforting to check in to our hotel room. Minutes later, zzzzzz. We let our slumber recharge us; tomorrow will be a busy day.

The FAQ for Plebe Parent Weekend provided by the Parent Communications Coordinator for West Point is our guiding light; plenty to do: tour the uniform factory, Jefferson Hall Library, academic open houses, Arvin Gym and PT demonstrations, along with an opportunity to tour Nate's room and the barracks. First up, a 6:30 AM appointment to tour Lusk Reservoir that is located next to Michie Stadium, all part of Nate's CH102 general chemistry course. His instructor asked the class to extend an invitation to family and friends. We gladly accept. The cadets gather outside the water treatment building, and the instructor welcomes us. A brisk morning, in the 20°Fs, and ice patches along the walkway.

"Please watch your step," he tells the group. And no sooner than he says these words, a cadet miscue unfolds right before our eyes and down goes the cadet. Thankfully, no injuries. The instructor goes on to explain the importance of Lusk as a water source for USMA and expands on other details of the academy grounds. He tells the group that the annual report of the Superintendent of USMA provide fantastic historical context of the changes and updates over the years. Then at Nate's expense, he adds that the volume of the reservoir is required knowledge of all Plebes. Here it comes.

"Nate, how many gallons in Lusk Reservoir?" the colonel asks.

"It has seventy-eight million gallons, sir," Nate sheepishly answers. Whew!

With a few hours until his next class, we decide to make a visit to Grant Hall Café to warm up, grab some coffee and a snack. We are all happy to be inside and out of the cold. Wow, no wind but the unforgiving twenty-degree temps are taking their toll. The warmth of being inside is welcomed no less than our excitement just to be here.

Nate, like all the other Plebes, continues to play the role of a tour guide for us. A visit into Thayer Hall makes its way on our places to see. A fast-paced walk leads us to the Thayer Award Room, one of the academy's crown jewels. The Sylvanus Thayer Award is presented to an outstanding citizen of the United States whose service and accomplishments in the national interests exemplify personal devotion to the ideals expressed in the West Point motto: "Duty, Honor, Country." The award room houses the portraits of every winner and features the likes of H. Ross Perot, Henry Kissinger, Tom Brokaw, and Neil Armstrong. On October 20, 2017, the Thayer Award was presented to former President George W. Bush. Only a few months into his West Point journey and Nate is attending an awards dinner and ceremony, with buzz and excitement in abundant supply, in Washington Hall sitting in the midst of a president. What an incredible opportunity and moment. In orderly fashion, the Olsavsky group departs Thayer Hall, and Cathy looks to take a repeat of a throwback picture on the walkaway next to the admissions building. Last January, this is where Sam told Nate he got an appointment to West Point. This time, standing next to Sam once again, Nate is dressed in gray—a cadet, a Plebe, a part of the Long Gray Line. *Snap!* Picture taken.

Spring break is in session at USMA and the Class of 2021 are the only ones on the grounds. Make no mistake, however, it's a beehive of activity. Moms and dads, grandparents, brothers and sisters, and friends, all trying to keep pace with their cadet, moving from location to location. For us, a quick stop in Eisenhower Hall and we make a beeline to the uniform factory. Yes, there are many options and sights to see while here for Plebe Parent Weekend, but the Cadet Uniform Factory (CUF) tour is a must-see. West Point's CUF is responsible for maintaining the traditional look of the Long Gray Line. It was formally brought into existence by an Act of Congress in 1878 and operates under regulation 10 USC4340. The amazing staff manufacture over sixty product lines from trousers to bathrobes to parkas to fitted full dress uniforms with forty-four gold-plated brass buttons. Dry cleaning, uniform-size adjustments, application of chevrons (the V-shape stripes indicating the cadet's rank), and service stripes and emblems are all part of a monthly personal services fee paid out of the cadet's salary. Yes, West Point cadets are paid a monthly salary based on their class year. Over their four years, cadets will pay $2,602.74 to the CUF for uniforms and support. Regardless of uniform type, the Corps of Cadets look impressive!

"Dad, Dad!" Sam is blurting out as he looks at me with sharp, piercing eyes.

Cathy adds on, "You just cut in line!"

"I didn't know," I say. "I was just following the tour guide's instruction." Call it dumb luck, but as we entered the doors to the CUF, there was room for four more in the next tour grouping. The waiting line was extended around the corner, and we stepped right in front of the greeting desk.

"Follow the line straight ahead." And off I went. The beauty of this was I don't think anyone noticed my misstep. Off we go. The guides talk about the materials used in all the gray uniforms, black parka, and other garments. A myriad of cutting, sewing, altering, and repairs are services provided to cadets. A flood of facts is highlighted for us, including where the wool comes from. Before the wool gets tailor-fitted to the Corps of Cadets, it grows out for a year on the back of sheep grazing in the Western US. And before Nate leaves to go to his next class, being the only cadet in attendance on our CUF tour, he's called out by the tour guide to model some of the uniform factory's exquisite tailoring. He stands there like a showpiece, more than happy to do his part for the crowd. For the crowd's part, I imagine they are taking in as much of West Point as possible and counting the hours, if not minutes, for the next rendezvous with their cadets. Like all much-anticipated events, the factory tour ends. There is a bonus to be had, though—gray-and-white swatches in the shapes of hearts and stars. Cathy picks up a few, and we check another place to visit off our list.

We have already walked over three miles and easily blend in to the highly organized and scheduled chaos on campus. People here, there, and everywhere. Nate rejoins us and parades us through the

Jefferson Library. The class ring display located in the library shows some of the oldest class rings from the academy's alumni. What a sight! Next stop is West Point's simulation center. Brotherly competition rears its head as Nate challenges Sam to the engagement skills trainer (EST) at the Department of Military Instruction's weapon-training event that supports weapons qualification and covers marksmanship and judgmental escalation-of-force exercises. Split-second decision-making determines the enemy from friendlies, and who do I shoot? Sam holds his own against his older brother, and it is clear to see Nate's Army training is taking root.

Our cadet tour guide, Nate, completes a show-and-tell of a few more places, including Academic Department Open Houses, before finishing out our afternoon on the academy grounds.

"We're going to go back to the hotel and freshen up," Cathy tells Nate.

We have a little free time before we need to meet up for the pinning ceremony in the courtyard.

At 6:00 PM, each company will be presented with the National Defense Service Medal and Ribbon by their TAC (tactical officer). Here we are. The courtyard is alive with cadets, organized chaos is in full swing as each company leader assembles their ranks. E-2 is nearly complete. Elsewhere in the vicinity, we hear "where is so-and-so?" and "the ceremony is going to start in a few minutes!"

Like all things West Point, everything comes together and E-2, A-1, C-3, I-4, etc., fall in line. Family members closely border the respective companies with their beloved Plebes. For most of these Plebes, this will be the first of many medals and ribbons to be displayed on their Army uniforms. The medal is a bronze medallion one and one-fourth inches in diameter. Shown on the front of medal beneath the words *National Defense* is an eagle with inverted wings perched on a sword and palm branch. The ribbon is one and three-eighths inches wide and has eleven stripes made up of four different colors: scarlet, white, blue, and yellow.

The TAC for E-2 finishes reading the award announcement and proceeds to hand out the medals to the E-2 Plebes. To my surprise, Nate walks over, and as we hug and congratulate him, he asks, "Dad, would you like to pin the medal on my uniform?" I find myself speechless, overcome with pride and holding back my excitement (and tears) to staidly say yes. That moment is permanently fixed in my mind. Shadows are scattered in every direction from the yellowed lighting being cast in the courtyard. Smiles and joyful congratulations can be heard throughout. Then Nate introduces us to one of his friends who is the guidon bearer for E-2.

"Dad, his family couldn't make it. Would you mind pinning his medal on?" Nate softly asks.

Without missing a beat, I turn to the young man and ask, "Can I do the honor of pinning your medal on?"

"Thank you, sir, yes," he responds.

In a matter of a few minutes, I have the unique opportunity to partake in a ceremony with not one but two West Point cadets to decorate the gray uniforms of these most deserving men. A true, sincere, and humbling act. Am I a proud dad? You bet! And I'm equally thrilled to lean in and help on this cold, bitter evening. Honestly, I would gladly pin each and every one of the Plebes from the Class of 2021. There is something about West Point—the atmosphere, history, the pride and accomplishments of these cadets that draws you in. As an insignificant outsider, I find myself connected to the magnificence and enormity of the mysterious call to duty embraced by these young men and women. Truly amazing.

Saturday-morning breakfast accommodations, 8:00 AM Washington Hall. We purchased tickets for $10 in advance to experience firsthand the pleasure of dining inside Washington Hall, the cadet mess. The tables, identified by company, are quickly filled by us and several hundred others looking for that special West Point moment with their Plebe. Nate gets us seated and, along with two other Plebes, begins to hand out plates, cups, silverware, napkins, and water. The flow of these items is reminiscent of the *I Love Lucy* chocolate factory where the conveyor belt speeds up and mayhem ensues. Breakfast is all business this morning with Nate. He is the acting platoon leader for E-2 and will be wearing the red sash, cadet parade tar bucket with feather plume, and officer sword entrusted to Firsties for the Plebe-Parent Review this afternoon. The Plebes will be conducting a practice run shortly after breakfast. The Plebe-Parent Review is a parade with only Plebes participating. The formation will consist of Plebes from each of the thirty-six companies in platoon-size formation (four by eight). The companies will march in order, Company A-1-Company I-4, led by the brigade staff. The color guard marches in between second and third regiments, and parents and guests can watch the parade from the sidewalks across from the superintendent's house—Quarters 100 and nearby on the snow-covered grass and roadway.

Nate gobbles down a few bites of scrambled eggs and finishes a drink of orange juice and leaves us to our own devices. He's heading out to check on E-2 and get the company assembled for the dry run. Not to be outdone, we make our way to the parade route and find a front-row spot almost directly across from Quarters 100. I jokingly make a comment that Supe Daddy (nickname for the USMA superintendent) will walk out the front door of Quarters 100 in a T-shirt with a coffee stain, disheveled hair, and wearing bunny slippers.

"Oh my goodness!" Cathy exclaims.

To our amazement, out walks the Supe in pajamas and a T-shirt and wearing a robe. He picks up a newspaper, looks across at the crowd, eyes right and left, and opens the door to return inside his house to a much warmer environment.

How funny is that? I think to myself.

Sore feet, aching calf muscles, and over-tensed neck and shoulders are the result of walking nearly eight miles yesterday in sub-freezing temperatures. We are among many, many others this frigid morning to watch the practice parade. There is nothing we won't do to catch a glimpse of our Plebes. Elbow to elbow and three, four, and five rows deep, the crowd comes to life as the Army band starts playing. Company by company, sounding off, "Ready, eyes right," platoons walk by the superintendent for inspection. Not too shabby for the not-so-new cadets.

At 2:00 PM, the scene repeats itself. This time, however, the morning crowd pales in comparison to the turnout for the formal parade. The superintendent and his entourage stand across from us, at the ready for the pass in review. The Army band harmoniously breaks out into John Philip Sousa's "The Washington Post."

The parade is underway and the pass in review of several companies of cadets marching past the reviewing stand for inspection only heightens our anticipation to see Nate leading his platoon.

Cathy has that innate (pun intended) talent, like most other moms here today, to pick out her child among the marching uniforms, all part of the very complex and often unexplained mother-child bond. And then...

"There's Nate!" she whispers to us. In perfect step, adorned in his full-dress gray jacket with white cross belts, rectangular shiny brass chest buckle, red sash and sword, and feather plume hat, Nate is introduced by the cadet announcer.

"Second platoon is led by Cadet Lieutenant Nathaniel Olsavsky from Friedens, Pennsylvania."

Nate flawlessly directs his eyes to the review stand, raises his right hand to a sharp salute and shouts, "Ready, eyes right. Ready, front!"

Sam's expert videography captures the moment and provides us a glimpse of how Nate, like a caterpillar radically transforming its body, eventually emerging as a butterfly, will one day morph from Plebe to Firstie.

Saturday night greets us with our first West Point formal event—the dressy occasion with the banquet in the cadet mess hall, followed by the hop to be held in Eisenhower Hall. Yes, this is not an informal event. It is a formal ball. We take our seats, and I think Cathy's nerves get the best of her as she spills a glass of water on the table. Not to worry, dinner is absolutely wonderful. And we make use of the helpful suggestion from the Plebe Parent Weekend FAQ: bring bubble wrap or socks. Why? To wrap your souvenir wine glasses. Today, these glasses reside in our china cabinet.

Spring break 2018 for the Class of 2021 is underway. No travel plans for Nate though. It's easy to see the physical and mental exhaustion on his face and his response to what's in store for the next week and a half before returning—rest, relax, eat, sleep, and do it all over again. Just like shampoo instructions, lather, rinse, repeat. Nate hasn't seen Hillary and Jacob's new house, so we revise our itinerary and make a stop in Chambersburg. We surprise Hill with a birthday cake, too, albeit belated. She's thrilled to see her brother, and they both get a nice sibling recharge from the visit.

"Good luck, Nate. You got this," Hillary says as we say our goodbyes and continue on with our travels on the last leg home. "Love you, buddy," she adds.

The early-March respite flashes by in the blink of an eye. And before we know it, we are once again making the three-hundred-plus mile, six-hour drive back to West Point. Along the way, we make a stop at Dick's Sporting Goods to buy a new pair of soccer cleats for Nate. The spring session of club soccer is starting up and on March 24 the team takes on the US Coast Guard Academy in New London, Connecticut. The away game sees the Black Knights notch up a win. And more importantly, simply spending some time outside the gates of West Point.

Volume 9 of Cadet Cody "Plebe Parent Weekend and Now Boxing" captures some of our favorite moments. Printed, folded, and the envelope is addressed, another volume mailed to hopefully provide a pick-me-up for Nate. And speaking of that elusive topic— no, not the cadet parka—I'm referring to b-o-x-i-n-g. Nate's boxing session is underway, and true to his word, he is not sharing one iota of information with us. The completion of his boxing commitment can't come soon enough for Cathy. For now, it's just a matter of wait and see. The perfect idiom for March holds its proverbial predictability, "March comes in like a lion, out like a lamb." The month's fierce cold weather ends on a much gentler note. April 2018 is here. Interestingly, the etymology behind the word *April* comes from the Latin word *aperire*, which means "to open." Like the arrival of spring, West Point sees the opening of many activities and things to do.

Near the top of the list is April 15, tax-filing due date. The West Point Tax Center prepares and files tax returns for cadets. This will be Nate's first tax return as a cadet and as the memorandum for the United States Corps of Cadets states, some of the items listed on the income tax return drop-off checklist should be discussed with their families. Cathy and I help review Nate's paperwork, and our young man is all smiles when he sees a windfall from both his federal and state returns. For his Pennsylvania personal tax return, income received for military service outside of Pennsylvania while on active duty as a member of the armed forces is not taxable compensation. Cha ching! West Point cadets are considered active-duty members of the military. Technically, according to AR600-20 Army Command Policy, cadets rank after commissioned and warrant officers, but before noncommissioned officers (NCOs).

At the top of the list, however, is none other than April 23, my birthday. Another late-evening drive on Friday, April 21, gets us to our destination for Saturday's much-anticipated Army versus Navy Club soccer game. And a pleasant way to spend my birthday weekend. The venue for today's rivalry match is Shea Stadium, located along the Hudson River. The stadium was named in honor of Richard Shea, a 1952 West Point graduate who was assigned to Korea following graduation and died in action on July 8, 1953, at Sokkogea, trying to repel Communist suicide attacks during the Korean conflict. He was posthumously awarded the Medal of Honor for wartime bravery.

The first half of this back-and-forth battle is reminiscent of last December's football game. A knockout, drag-out game, and Nate has paid the price. In a defensive struggle for ball possessions near the midfield sideline, Nate gets tripped and his knee and elbow are bloodied and scraped up pretty good. Not so long ago, he was throwing himself in at 110 percent in the very same way during his senior year high school games. Navy capitalizes on a few Army miscues and takes a 1–0 lead into halftime. Navy is just too good, too on top of their game this afternoon; they turn in a few more goals and claim victory in a shoot-out over the Black Knights. Disappointing? No, not really. We are among only a small group of spectators in the sun-reflecting bleachers this afternoon and get more than our share of Army-Navy team photos. Pretty cool.

We make the most out of the afternoon in an all-encompassing catch-up conversation over a relaxing dinner for the four of us— Cathy, Nate, Sam, and me. Time is always set on hyperdrive at West Point, whether for Nate and his incredibly demanding schedule or simply how one event jumps to the next, how one day blends into the following. This holds true for all of us. Sunday morning brunch sees us at the Park Restaurant in Highland Falls. Unlike previous stops here, this meal comes with a surprise for me! Cathy hands me an envelope while Nate and Sam each give me a wrapped gift. I honestly didn't see any of these things in Cathy's shoulder bag. Tomorrow is my birthday! As I get older, the birthday celebrations begin to blend into one another. But that doesn't make them any less special or meaningful. My high school friend and college roommate was a huge Rush, the Canadian rock band, fan known for their complex musical compositions that drew heavily on fantasy and philosophy. He listened to them nonstop. The Rush song "The Garden" comes to mind as I relish in this birthday moment:

> The measure of a life is a measure of love and respect
> So hard to earn, so easily burned,
> In the fullness of time
> A garden to nurture and protect.

A beautiful song that reminds us to hold on to the real things that matter in our lives. Life needs constant maintenance. Our family, now with Cody, is solid and strong and we hold life's real things close to our hearts.

The card from Cathy warms my heart. I unwrap Sam's gift, a gray T-shirt with Top Dad printed on the front. A humorous tie-in to one of our family favorites, *Top Gun*, featuring Tom Cruise. And last but not least, I open Nate's gift—a book, a signed copy of Alan Alda's (Hawkeye) *If I Understood You, Would I Have This Look on My Face*.

"I got it when he spoke at the Modern War Institute Round Table," Nate tells me.

And the Top Dad T-shirt, what can I say? Priceless. Two years later and I'm still proudly wearing it.

Last up on our list of things to do before we say our goodbyes is a stop to see the new visitor's center. The Frederic V. Malek West Point Visitor's Center opened on December 4, 2017, and is home to twenty-seven thousand square feet of displays and exhibits (and another Army West Point gift shop). Malek was a 1959 graduate of the United States Military Academy and a successful businessman and was instrumental in the vision and process to build the state-of-the-art facility. Exhibits include a full-scale cadet barracks room, a cadet uniform room, cadet daily life, academic fields of endeavor, and the admissions process. And the most picturesque sight? Entering the center places you under the view of the cadet hat toss with photographs of Ulysses S. Grant, John Joseph Pershing, Douglas MacArthur, Dwight David Eisenhower, and Omar Nelson Bradly looking on. Wow!

Sunday evening text message to Nate, 8:00 PM: "Hi, Nate, we just got home, all good. We had a great time. Miss and love you bunches. You got this."

Like March, the month of April is on full throttle. Nate's friend talks him into volunteering for the West Point Scoutmaster's Council Camporee scheduled for April 27–29 at the Lake Frederick Recreation area located seven miles from the USMA. Sure, Nate thinks, why not? A chance to get away from the familiar scenes on post and get outdoors. More than six thousand Boy and Girl Scouts, Venture Crews, and Civil Air Patrol cadets, along with nearly one thousand volunteers, are planning to engage with West Point staff, faculty, and cadets. Army weaponry, wilderness survival, litter carry, first aid, knot tying, camouflage, and how to march are the orders of the day. And this year, Nate shares over and over again all it is doing is raining. Wet, damp clothes and mud are in abundant supply. But the bright spot readily shows at the badge stations where these young boys and girls try to collect as much West Point cadet brass as possible for bragging rights. Luckily, Nate and the other cadets are bunked in cabins, so unlike the scouts, they avoid the downpours, flooded tents, and rain-soaked sleeping bags. The weekend-long camporee ends on multiple high notes as the scouts, with smiles and eyes opened as wide as the wingspan of the mosquitos they've battled, observe mock demonstrations of military operations such as air assault missions with helicopters, a large bonfire, and a military review parade involving the USMA leadership.

Plebe year is rapidly approaching the finish line. Every step along the way, our newest family member Cody has lovingly taken to us. He has a passion for his squeaky toys and tennis ball and enjoys being held tightly for a nap. It will be cool to see his reaction again to Nate opening the front door when he comes home for his short summer break.

Too bad Cody won't be able to see Nate all decked out in his India white uniform. Like so many other firsts for the Class of 2021, the India whites are yet another new uniform issue to add to their ever-growing cadet wardrobe. Their first opportunity to wear them comes at the completion of cadet field training (CFT) at Camp Buckner in July. This is when they make the transition from Plebe to "Pluck" to Yearling (Yuk) and celebrate at a formal known as the Camp Illumination Hop.

Another follow-up doctor's appointment for Sam to check on his progress and his orthopedic surgeon gives him more than great news; she calls him her perfect patient. And clears him for all activities, including soccer, when school starts in the fall. Hard to believe it has been over a year since his spinal fusion surgery. To say we are blessed is an understatement.

Blessings come in all shapes and sizes. Today, May 9, Cathy receives two pictures from Nate—individual and group boxing photos. Nate provides some details on a Sunday-evening call. He had his *bell* rung a few times and saw others with bloody noses, cadets dropped with concussions, and an assortment of other injuries. Luckily, he made it through relatively unscathed. Yes, boxing is now history! We all breathe a sigh of relief!

The last of the cadet academic activities are winding down, and the TEE schedules are set in place. One week of final exams to power through, and Nate, along with his friends and the other '21 Plebes, will have one academic year under their belts.

More good news. Nate lets us know he has been invited to an awards ceremony to recognize cadets' outstanding academic achievement in mathematics. It is widely known that the math program at the United States Military Academy is extremely challenging, so we are thrilled to hear of Nate's accomplishment. He tells us it is a relatively brief event to recognize students for their exemplary performance throughout their four years at West Point and those that achieved the highest average in math courses during the 2018 spring term. Nate sends us a text with a picture of him holding a black two-sleeved envelope, smiling away: "Certificate of Commendation presented to Nathaniel Olsavsky by the Department of Mathematical Sciences in Recognition of Outstanding Achievement as 'Top Gun' in MA255, Advanced Multivariable Calculus, Spring 2018."

There is little rest for the weary. Nevertheless, Nate does find a few days of R & R in between his last exam and the start of his summer training. Following a trip to Ocean City, Maryland, with friends, he has some fun in the sun and enjoys the all-you-can-eat seafood buffet. He begins the infamous Zero Day on May 26 for the Sabalauski Air Assault School. The intense ten-day, three-phase journey is led by instructors, known to the cadet trainees as Black Hats, from the 101st Airborne Division from Fort Campbell, Kentucky.

Nate is among 180 candidates who start Zero Day with a two-mile run in combat uniform within a time of 18:00 and successful negotiation of the Marne Obstacle Course overlooking the Hudson River. The three phases, each lasting three days, are broken into combat assault phase, sling load phase, and rappel phase where the cadets can be viewed from the patio at Cullum Hall or the roof parking lot at Thayer Hall.

Not to miss anything, we make the trip to West Point to watch Nate rappelling from the forty-foot tower and a UH60 Black Hawk helicopter. We watch in awe from the Thayer Hall rooftop as the candidates, group by group, jump in the helicopters, climb in elevation with the constant reverberation of rotor blade noise, then methodically make them repel out of the Black Hawk. It is hard to describe the sights and sounds; but the feelings—those patriotic, proud, raw parental suite of emotions—crash over us in swells. That is why we are here. To be a part of Nate's successful completion of training, marked with the culmination of a twelve-mile road march with assault pack and inspection of his equipment—all within three hours or he fails.

"Hey, guys," Nate greets us on a call. "I passed."

"That's great," Cathy replies. "We're so proud of you." Out of 180 candidates, 131 make it through successfully.

On another beautiful, warm, and welcoming day this Saturday, June 9, 2018, we have the honor of attending the air assault graduation ceremony at Trophy Point. The commandant is the class guest speaker. We are among a relatively small group in attendance, but everyone is beaming with smiles as far as the eyes can see. Even more so as the Black Shirts conclude the ceremony by awarding each candidate with the coveted Air Assault Badge, an oxidized silver badge consisting of a helicopter superimposed upon a pair of stylized wings displayed and curving inward. So much hard work, sweat, pain, and discipline in that badge. Now similar to the presentation of the National Defense Service Medal in March, I rise from the ranks of the ordinary to being brought into the esoteric and arcane matter of pinning the Air Assault Badge on Nate's uniform. Another event that transcends time and space. There is a quote from an anonymous pen that says, "To be in your children's memories tomorrow, you have to be in their lives today." Definitely words to live by. I clasp the pin and Nate displays his achievement, standing tall, wide-brimmed smile. *Click!* Cathy captures the memory!

It has been a whirlwind schedule for Nate since the Firsties graduation on May 26, 2018. The Chairman of the Joint Chiefs of Staff, Marine Corps, Gen. Joe Dunford, was the commencement speaker. Cathy and I watched from the comfort of our living room. The general's words strike deep as he addresses the Class of 2018, "You chose to join an Army at war." He goes on to tell them, "Character, competence, courage, and commitment is part of the sticker price of being an Army leader. After West Point, you get no credit for that. It's a given. When you check into your units, your soldiers will simply want to know that you will lead from the front and you will put their interests ahead of your own."

All this training goes to laying the foundations for leading from the front, fast-moving pieces which are par for the course for a West Point cadet. And just like that, Nate's ten-day break following air assault is coming to an end. Sam and Nate take in a movie, a few stops at Taco Bell, and cast a few lines trout fishing. Our boys, loving brothers to the core, shorten those lines of separation. Yeah, Cody's fun-loving ways and lightning-fast sprints in the backyard, chasing birds, add to the enjoyment of simply being home.

Sam captures many of these whimsical occasions and volume 10 of *The Adventures of Cadet Cody* shows a canine yawn of biblical proportions. The pic is outstanding in its own right, but how Sam times the moment and sight leaves me scratching my head, how does he do it? So cool! Not to be outdone, I follow up with a pic of two deer leisurely walking through the backyard. Almost as if they know they are being watched, a brief pause, two deliberate stares with heads-up, saying, "Take your picture already." I oblige while Cody misses out on the entire event. He is napping.

The prelude to Yearling year is underway as the plucks report to Camp Buckner for CFT. When the academic year ended, the Plebe Class of 2021 became Yearlings. Their actual promotion to cadet corporals will be when they complete all summer training requirements which comes at the completion of CFT.

Nate finished getting his cadet-packing list together while on break. Always something to prep. Bug spray, 550 cord, camo face paint, map protector, red lens flashlight, and two dozen more items are on the list.

Buckner offers little in the way of accommodations. Honestly, it looks like a scene out of a WWII training camp—dirt roads, metal-skinned bays, overgrown trees, and a view of the lake. Cathy diligently and faithfully keeps up with writing Nate letters. Mine are fewer and farther apart and the Cadet Cody highlights are dwindling as well. Nate sends us a postcard with a few highlights from CFT. Two of his bunkmates are soldiers with the Hellenic Army from Greece. I'm not sure if they were part of the group that found the rattlesnake inside their bay. Nate said they were instructed about wildlife protecting and the surrounding woodlands. So someone corralled the snake into a small pan can and released it outside. Really, Nate? You could have left the snake part out of the postcard and spared Mom the anxiety. We also hear about the laundry facilities. Or rather the lack of them. However, Buckner isn't about cleaning ACUs.

Newly promoted Firsties fill the officer positions, and much of the training focuses on small-unit infantry tactics. Advanced rifle marksmanship and assault course, confidence obstacle course, combat skills, Recondo Day, OPFOR (opposing forces) and small unit weapons balance out the summer training regimen. OPFOR pits the Yearlings against an opposing force made up of regular Army training unit soldiers along with the help of Cows and Firsties.

Nate shares details how his company fought hard but was no match for the opposing enemy forces. To add insult to injury, he also fell, and his chin caught the butt end of his rifle, resulting in a nasty cut. The medics looked him over and said the gash could probably use a couple of stitches, but he opted for the butterfly bandage. I'm not sure how this fits in, but the medic covered the butterfly bandage with two colorful SpongeBob Band-Aids. Yeah, I think they were messing with him a bit. Nate said he heard laughter as they walked away, so even the Army has a sense of humor. Go figure.

CFT is winding down. The cadets take on the water confidence course (or slide for life) in their final days of training. The obstacle is comprised of two phases—the slide for life and the beam walk-rope drop. The goal: build confidence and beat back any fear of heights and water. A tough task by any measure but these cadets come through. Nate tells us there was a light drizzle on his training day and cadets were having difficulty holding on, so they had to shut down the slide for the day. Safety first.

On July 28, 2018, the Class of 2021 completes CFT requirements with a 7.15 mile run back from Camp Buckner as the Class of 2022 begins its final phase of CBT with their march out to Buckner. The run back to post is led by the company that had the highest cumulative Recondo score. You guessed it! Nate's company takes the lead. And for us, we're here to watch the awards and promotion ceremony on the camp parade grounds with hundreds of other anxious and excited families.

The cadets march on to the grounds in crisp order in front of the crowds overfilling the bleachers. The shaded seats begin to be overtaken by the morning sun, and beads of sweat are racing down the channel of my spine. My forehead and face are dripping as well. It is sweltering outside, and we begin to see some of the effects from the oppressive heat. One of the cadets in the very first row collapses.

Then another cadet drops. And another cadet further back falls to the ground. Surprisingly, none of the fellow cadets to the left, right, or behind these "heat cats" (heat casualties) break formation to help. Not to worry. Situations such as these are planned for, and we quickly see medics coming to their aid. A cursory evaluation then the dropped cadets are assisted to the rear of the formation. Most likely dehydration or heat exhaustion. I see several cases of bottled water in the distance. Thank goodness.

West Point training events are typically named after former cadets who have paid the ultimate sacrifice. This cadet field training promotion ceremony was named in honor of US Army Captain Scott Pace, USMA 2005. Captain Pace was on a rescue mission in Afghanistan in 2011. He was in command of a patrol helicopter when he and his copilot were dispatched to save soldiers who were under fire. Sadly, the helicopter was hit by gunfire and went down in the desert, killing both Captain Pace and his copilot. However, thanks to Pace's brave, courageous, and selfless efforts and sacrifice, all the soldiers on the ground were able to escape alive.

The Task Force Pace CFT graduation ceremony was honored to have the Pace family in attendance. Mr. Patrick Pace spoke of his son and the sacrifices he made while offering words of encouragement, of pride, and congratulations to the newly promoted Yearlings.

I remember Mr. Pace speaking directly to the cadets and kindly asking them, perhaps a friendly request in its simplest form, that the cadets "please take the time to write home." Send mom and dad a handwritten letter, skip the texts and e-mails, and put pen to paper. Such a simple, pure, and heartfelt message. And it strikes home. It's like he's been talking to Nate all this time. And Cathy as well. The exchange of letters is a two-way street.

There are many teary-eyed faces among those here today. The hard reality is that America's sons and daughter, our children, have committed their talents and their love of God, country, and family to place themselves in harm's way.

As the ceremony nears completion, people begin to point to the sky and heads look up into the blue sky. Sam quietly says, "Look, an eagle!" He pulls his camera out to take a picture. A beautiful sight, a bald eagle soaring high above the cadets taking advantage of thermals and updrafts. The bald eagle is our national symbol and appears on currency, official documents, flags, public buildings and is used in the military and by government agencies.

Today, the appearance of the bald eagle represents the sacrifice of Captain Pace and the accomplishments of the Class of 2021 Yearling cadets. Coincidence? Perhaps. I am inclined to believe that our heavenly Father sent this beautiful bird of flight to offer comfort, strength, and peace of mind for all of us.

We have come full circle from that early Sunday, July 2, 2017, morning departure from our home. Many of our concerns have dissipated. The unknowns have faded. We have been warmly welcomed and lovingly stitched into the Long Gray Line extended families' fabric of pride. We've had our ups and downs, laughed and cried and missed phone calls, and have been surprised with unexpected notes from our Plebe. That was yesterday and those were last year's events. Nate is a Plebe no more. The close of the last twelve months is a time for reflection. It is also a time to look forward to the promise of what is to come and staying strong. What does the future at West Point hold for our cadet? What does the future have in store for us?

CHAPTER 7

These Forty-Seven Months Are Flying By!

IT SEEMS LIKE those July summer evenings were days ago. I didn't have a care in the world. The sounds and sights of fireworks were nonstop—M-80s and firecrackers going off, sparklers being lit and waved by people of all ages, bottle rockets aimed above the tree lines and colors of red, white, and blue blanketing every town, village, and city, large and small, across the country. The time was July 4, 1976, and the Unites States of America was celebrating the two-hundred-year bicentennial anniversary of the adoption of the Declaration of Independence.

Now decades later, I see how the words of that document are piercing our family with so much more meaning: *"And for the support of this Declaration, with a firm reliance on the protection of divine Providence, we mutually pledge to each other our lives, our fortunes and our sacred Honor."* This is Nate's calling.

As an easygoing, happy-go-lucky twelve-year-old, me, and my neighborhood friends saw our simple small-town lives revolve around catching fireflies at night, looking at constellations and counting stars, swatting mosquitos, gathering enough players for a pick-up baseball game, fishing, and playing red rover and hide-and-seek under the streetlights. Perhaps I had scant thoughts that someday, maybe someday, I'd find myself married, I'd be a father. Those are memories from several lifetimes ago. Fast forward to today. Sam and Nate share the same affinity in my taste in music from those bygone days. And Hillary, well, she has that same streak of stubbornness like her old man.

Jean-Baptiste Alphonse Karr, French novelist, said, "The more that things change, the more they stay the same." How true. I can't help but break out into a smile when I hear songs from Blue Oyster Cult, Boston, Electric Light Orchestra, Kiss, Journey, Cheap Trick, Fleetwood Mac, the Doobie Brothers, and many other classic rock groups blasting on the boys' playlists. It cracks me up when they both blare "Brandy (You're a Fine Girl)" by Looking Glass from their Bose speakers.

In February 2008, for Nate's ninth birthday, Cathy bought concert tickets for him and me to see The Machine: The Pink Floyd Experience, a tribute band at the Arcadia Theatre in Windber, Pennsylvania. He was definitely the youngest fan in attendance! Since then, Nate, Sam, Cathy, and I have seen Kansas, Tom Petty and The Heartbreakers, Peter Frampton, and Lynyrd Skynyrd perform. I feel like there's a different ring to the music these days. Maybe the sounds are the same, but the way I hear things and see things have changed. The effects of the passing of many seasons, I guess.

Here we are, more than forty years later from those fun-filled summer bicentennial days of 1976, and I find myself yet looking ahead once again. One thing is clear, I'm an older man. Three kids, all mature, on their way to being successful, and most importantly, they are polite, caring, and respectful individuals. Looking ahead, we wonder, *What's in store for Hillary, Sam, and our up-and-coming US Army officer?*

Reorgy (reorganization) week for the first semester of the 2018–2019 academic year is underway for Nate. It is mid-August where cadets are returning from summer vacation and summer training, and the cadet cadre are preparing the Class of 2022. A hectic week with company assignments and academic changes and various training briefs.

Nate sends us a good morning message and tells us that he's going to the Supe's Academic Awards ceremony at Robinson

Auditorium in Thayer Hall. The ceremony highlights the academic achievements from the spring 2018 semester with the awarding of the Superintendent's Award for Excellence and Achievement and the Distinguished Cadet Award. Cadets earn the award for excellence by demonstrating outstanding performance in all three programs: academic, physical, and military. The top 5 percent of each class earns the award, which is a gold star encircled by a wreath. The Distinguished Cadet Award goes to cadets who earn a quality point average of 3.67 or higher, and they receive a gold star. The top 15 percent awardees of each class receives a gold wreath.

"Hey, guys, I got called up on stage at the Supe's award ceremony this morning," Nate messages. Included in his text is a pic of two pins: a gold star encircled by a wreath and a gold wreath. Cathy and I look at each other and quietly, proudly, and excitedly smile from ear to ear. Our Yearling has found his groove. West Point and the Army's discipline and unyielding structure all suit Nate quite well.

Never being afraid to try something new, Nate surprises us with his latest foray—the West Point Spirit Band. "Yeah, I want to take a break from soccer," he tells us. Nate's roommate, who also plays the war tuba for the Spirit Band, convinces Nate to join the band. There's a spot for a mellophone player. And simultaneously, Cathy and I look at each other and ask, "What's a mellophone?" A quick Google search provides us with the answer. A mellophone is a two- or three-valve brass instrument similar to a French horn. Pretty cool! Bring on the music!

Cathy sets up the TV to record all of Army's football games that will be televised on CBS Sports Network. Now rather than focusing on the play-by-play game action, we see ourselves talking to the cameramen and asking them to zoom in on the band. Anything for a glimpse of our cadet.

The band affords Nate a lot of opportunities throughout the autumn season to get off West Point grounds. A trip to the Pentagon, Washington, DC, is a highlight leading up to the Army-Navy game on December 8, 2018, where we enjoy watching Army extending their streak with a 17–10, nail-biting win over Navy. To top off the season, Nate enjoys a pre-Christmas road trip to Fort Worth, Texas, where Army took on Houston in the Armed Forces Bowl played on December 22, 2018. The Black Knights shattered all kinds of NCAA bowl records in a 70–14 blowout!

On the home front, fall soccer season is in full swing for Sam as he enters his junior high school year. Beyond words to see him active, running around, and back to normal physical activities. However, Sam is a soccer-injury magnet. Last year, in preseason camp, he fractured his wrist, and now he sends us a pic of blood streaming down his nose, covering his face. Luckily, it was just a cut on the bridge, and yes, he continues on, smiling away and taking it all in stride. Thank goodness.

The changing of the seasons is once again upon us. A cornucopia of autumn colors blankets the hillsides and valley, at home, and along the Hudson Valley. Cathy plans a Sunday-afternoon excursion for Sam, her, and me to take in a scenic train ride in Romney, West Virginia. The Potomac Eagle Scenic Railroad takes us on a journey along the south branch of the Potomac River through an amazing and visually striking gorge home to many American bald eagles. We share our photo-op moments—eagles flying overhead, the crisp river, and the colorful trees—with Hillary and Nate. What a cool way to spend several hours on a Sunday afternoon, nowhere to be and no time to keep. Although separated, we are five; we are family, plus one—Cody!

The waning days of October hits our family, the parish family of St. Peter's, and the extended Somerset community with sad news. After a valiant, long-fought battle with cancer, Father Daniel O'Neill, pastor of St. Peter's and our dear friend, passed away. Nate had a special relationship with Father O'Neill, so Cathy and I discuss how best to break the news to him. We reach out to his chain of command and also contact the chaplains at Most Holy Trinity Catholic Chapel. Both indicate it's best for us to share the news with Nate, and they let us know that they'll follow up with him afterward to check in. The West Point family at work.

We send Nate a text message to give us a call when he has some free time. Not long after, our phone rings.

"Hi, what's going on?" he asks in a reserved manner. He knows something is up.

"Hi, Nate," Cathy says. "We wanted to let you know Father O'Neill passed away today."

There's silence, a sigh, and we hear a few sobs and sense some tears. Parents know. We comfort him in our conversation and tell him we contacted his TAC and Most Holy Trinity and that they'll probably be reaching out to check in. We'll be up next weekend, November 3, for the Air Force football game, we repeat.

"Hang in there, Nate. Remember you can call us anytime, day or night," we tell him. "We love you."

The joys of life and the reality of coming to terms with our mortality and acceptance of death, the realization that everyone's days are numbered, go hand in hand. One knows not the day or hour; we've heard this many times at Mass. Is this a wake-up call for our family? Not really. I see time after time where our kids find the good in the world, they look at the wonder and beauty that surrounds them, and they use that as momentum to fuel their lives and cherish the simplest of things. We aren't afraid to cry or laugh or argue or find agreement where it may not be readily found. Yes, these tears will pass.

The October days pass by and November sees our cadet highlighted in West Point's *Pointer View* magazine. November 11, 2018, marks the one hundredth anniversary of the World War I armistice. West Point put out a call to the Corps of Cadets, asking who may have had family ties to WWI. The *Pointer View* November 15, 2018, edition provides a fitting tribute to the historical occasion: "Current Cadets follow in the sacrifices made by their grandparents in World War I" written by Brandon O'Connor. O'Connor writes:

> World War I officially ended 100 years ago Sunday. Three generations have passed between the American Soldiers who fought and died upon the battlefields of France and cadets learning to be leaders in the Army at West Point. Although they never met, cadets whose ancestors fought in the Great War have still found inspiration from

their forefathers' service as they prepare to begin their own.

The article continues:

Class of 2021 Cadet Nathaniel Olsavsky carries his families' legacy with him every day. His middle name Joseph harkens back to his paternal great-grandfather Joseph Liko who served as a private in the Army during World War I. More than 130 years after he was born and 100 years after he served in the Army, Liko's story has encouraged multiple generations to follow in his footsteps and join the Army. "This connection definitely inspired me to join the Army and pursue an appointment from West Point," Olsavsky said. "The family history of how both my grandfather and great-grandfather served in the Army, and the stories of hard times and uncertainty in the world attracted me to serve in the Army. My initial desire came from my grandfather who served in World War II and the Korean War, and I later became interested to learn more about my great-grandfather." That connection to his family and the man whose name he carries have only deepened during his time at West Point, Olsavsky said. As he spends his days with fellow cadets who have chosen to serve and who are willing to sacrifice their lives for America, Olsavsky said he draws comfort from the stories of his great-grandfather and grandfather as he knows he is sharing "the same camaraderie that my great-grandfather experienced."

"The 100-year anniversary reminds me of all the men and women, from all different backgrounds who gave their all, some making the ultimate sacrifice," Olsavsky said. "They became a true part of something larger than themselves and dedicated their lives to their love of country. The call to service to our great nation is the same as it was 100 years ago, connecting the present with the future."

And November delivers a second surprise to us. Nate asks if he can bring a friend home for Thanksgiving.

"Absolutely, that sounds great!" we tell Nate. "Your friends are always welcome to join us."

Jim, my brother-in-law, and I meet the duo at mile marker 219 westbound on I-80 on Wednesday evening. It's a planned rest stop for the Western Pennsylvania West Point Parents' Club cadet bus. And before you know it, I'm pulling into the driveway and the boys are greeted to warm hugs and kisses from Cathy. The fragrant aroma of Thanksgiving is already in the air—pumpkin and apple pies are hot out of the oven and all the other preparations await our early morning wake up call. But for now, it's pepperoni pizza and buffalo chicken dip for the boys. Cody takes an immediate liking and quickly realizes that this new affection rewards him with a few tidbits of pizza crust. Yep, he's fitting right in! And Nate and his friend fill their free time on break—a Black Friday shopping excursion and a trip to the rifle range to practice pistol shooting.

And just like that, Thanksgiving leads the way to December and the Army-Navy game, a fun-filled weekend in Philadelphia with friends, tailgating in perfect weather, and, most importantly, another Army win, 17–10. Go Army! Beat Navy!

The best part of this holiday season, however, is getting the green light from Hillary and Jacob to share their wonderful news with family and friends. Yes, you guessed right! A new addition to the family. We're going to be grandparents in the New Year! And Nate and Sam will soon be uncles with Hillary's June 2019 delivery date.

A few months pass by and our joy and growing anticipation fades as sad news rips through our family at the very beginning of April. We are devastated. We tragically lose my brother, Tom. The ten little Indians are now nine. Tom was the fourth youngest among the ten siblings. He was a US Army reservist.

One week before the shocking and unfathomable events of September 11, 2001, Tom received his notification that he was officially assigned to the Retired Reserve, having dutifully served twenty years in the US Army Reserve. He enjoyed every minute of it. Our brother was a proud and faithful servant to his country. His love of God, country, and family was unquestionable and his commitment to the 464th Chemical Brigade was commendable. Uncle Tommy hung up his last uniform as a Master Sergeant—Thomas J. Olsavsky, Signal Support Chief with seven longevity stripes slanted down his left sleeve.

I clearly remember when Tommy called Nate in early June 2017 to wish him well prior to going to West Point for R-Day. Well wishes is one way to describe the conversation. Tommy's vernacular was colorful, to say the least. Nate was chuckling as Uncle Tommy dropped a few f-bombs, telling him that Army basic training was a "mind game and the drill instructors were there to f——k with them." Too funny. Tommy ended the conversation by saying that he was so f——ing proud of him. "You're going to be an officer!" he said. "Your grandfather would be thrilled!"

Dear brother and Uncle Tommy, you are truly missed.

Like all of life's curveballs that are thrown at us, time begins to take the sting out of our pain and loss. Time does, indeed, heal all wounds, and our time takes us into the celebration of Easter. Unlike last year, our plans take us to West Point on April 20 to spend the Easter weekend with Nate and his roommate. Cathy makes reservations at the Residence Inn in Fishkill, New York, and our weekend is set. First up, meet the boys Friday evening after their classes finish, grab dinner, and relax.

Nate and I wake up early Saturday morning and drive to the Pennsylvania Department of Transportation Driver's License Center in Milford, Pennsylvania, about an hour away from Fishkill. His license expired in February and getting a new one has been on the to-do list. Check! Next up, a shopping jaunt. We hit a number of stores at the Poughkeepsie Galleria Mall and buy Nate a new wardrobe for his three-week end-of-semester Academic Individual Advanced Development (AIAD) training in Rochefort, France. Rochefort has an important Air Force base and two specialized military and technical schools. What an incredible opportunity. Nate will study French at one of France's military language schools and explore a new culture during this time away from USMA. His plans are set, and he'll depart shortly after the graduation ceremony for the West Point Class of 2019 cadets. But at this very minute, he's spending mom and dad's money on a wardrobe upgrade to make him stand out as a sharply dressed man. Yep. New shoes, shorts, slacks, and shirts. He'll fit in just fine, *oui oui!* The Oakley-polished white sunglasses are the icing on the cake.

Saturday evening comes quickly, and the boys are working hard, catching up on homework assignments, faces deep in the pages of their textbooks. Cathy and I prep for a home-cooked Easter Sunday meal in the kitchenette. On the menu: honey baked ham, kielbasa, deviled eggs, sweet potato casserole, green beans and buttered corn, rolls, and brownies and chocolate chip cookies. Oh yeah, they're going to get the royal treatment from Cathy.

"Happy Easter!" Cathy greets the boys and lets them know that the Easter bunny made a surprise visit at some point during the night and delivered three baskets filled with peanut butter meltaways, jelly beans, marshmallow peeps, chocolate-covered pretzels, and foil-wrapped chocolate eggs. The smiles from the boys are resounding confirmation that this little touch of home away from home is warmly welcomed—a glaring success!

Everyone dresses in their traveling Sunday best outfits, and we attend Easter mass at St. Mary, Mother of the Church, in Fishkill. Young and old alike are dressed in a myriad of pastel colors, lighting up the church pews on this blessed day, recognizing and acknowledging what Jesus Christ said, over and over, that we shouldn't be afraid. Jesus showed us perfect love. And yet our human frailties overtake us parents. We often dwell and fear on what the future may have in store for our children, particularly our second lieutenants in the making. Where will Nate and his friends be stationed? Will they be placed in harm's way? Will they be happy? Natural feelings for all of us, I imagine. For now, we focus on the present, and our attention turns to the picturesque sight of the place settings on the table and the hot, aromatic food coming out of the oven. What a sight!

"Be careful. Watch the lid. It's hot," Cathy tells me. Too late. "Ouch!" I grimace aloud as I burn three of my fingers on the pot lid. Cathy and the boys relish in my miscue and can't help but laugh at my expense as I briefly run my fingers under cold water. Then like a scene out of Bill Murray's *Groundhog Day*, I reach over to take the lid off the smaller pot, and yikes!

"I can't believe I did that!" I say to the continuing laughter. Oh well, nothing serious as I humbly enjoy the delicious feast laid out before us. The boys indulge in a second helping, and the conversation moves on to the last item on our "things to do" list—a visit to the Walkway Over the Hudson State Historic Park. Cathy has been talking about coming here for a while, and finally, the right time is here. The park provides access to the Hudson River's breathtaking landscape with 1.28-mile-long deck, 212 feet above the river's surface. The boys oblige for several photo-op moments, and Nate's roommate's mom is thrilled to see the pics and even more pleased that we *adopted* him for the Easter weekend. The West Point family of families never thinks twice about taking in one of their own and helping others.

Back home, and after a few months of living in a state of emotional highs and lows, a return to normalcy pleasantly arrives with Sam going to Somerset's junior-senior high school prom. Sam joins a close group of friends on May 10, 2019, wearing a sleek, cobalt-blue tuxedo by Sarno & Sons. Our eleventh-grade guy is looking sharp! And we share all the photos with Hillary and Nate; everyone is in agreement; Sam is one handsome young man! And a capable handyman too. Sam and I take a Sunday afternoon in the first week of June to replace the original dishwashing machine in the kitchen with a new Frigidaire Gallery model to match our oven and microwave. Like all my home improvement projects, a relatively simple plug-and-play replacement DIY project turns into several hours as I struggle to make the water line connection. But we succeed!

Shortly into the month of June, Nate departs JFK Airport in New York City and lands at Charles de Gaulle Airport in Paris, France. Several connecting train rides later has him and a few other West Point cadets arriving in Rocheforte. His AIAD is underway. And by the look of the pictures and text messages he's sending us, France is treating him pretty well.

The only thing topping Nate's adventures comes on June 8, 2019. At 10:47 PM, Noah Daniel enters the world at twenty-one inches, seven pounds and eight ounces. Hillary and Jacob are proud, happy, totally thrilled parents to a healthy, bubbly, and energetic baby boy. And Cathy and me? Well, we decide on our grandparent names: Gramma and PawPaw! Cathy takes care of Sam's and Nate's new status as well. Prior to Nate leaving for France, she custom-made black T-shirts with white lettering, *Promoted to Uncle*. Sam wears his shirt to the hospital when we visit Hillary and Noah for the first time. She lights up! The smile jumps off her face when she sees Nate's pic from the beach—sun, sand, and surf in the background, with him proudly bearing the message of his newly declared promotion. Pretty cool stuff! Proud parents, proud grandparents, and proud uncles. And we jokingly refer to Stella and Remi as Noah's older sister and brother, and Cody now carries the moniker of Uncle Cody.

Speaking of rank, on June 28, Cathy and I sign up and volunteer for Mock R-Day as fresh-faced cadets. The US Military Academy relies each year on a platoon of volunteers to help choreograph Reception Day and what happens after the infamous sixty-second farewell in Eisenhower Hall. More than two hundred civilians, ages twelve and up, reported for R-Day for 2019's practice to help Firsties and Cows iron out the kinks in the details from equipment distribution, saluting, and marching instructions. A West Point cadet I am not! Immediately after walking out of the serenity and quietness of Ike Hall, it begins. Cadets wearing the red sash, with daggers glaring from their eyes, screaming, yelling, and barking orders. Holy cow! Intimidating? You bet! We're separated into groups of ten to fifteen people, and as luck would have, I get assigned to E-2. Cathy is assigned to a different company, but we cross paths as company by company of cadets are marched between the time-weathered buildings and the courtyard. So much walking, if you can even call it that. More like an out-of-sync, fast-paced trot. And then I see Nate with several other cadets at the corner of one of the buildings. They're enjoying the coolness from the shade and chuckling as the volunteer wannabees are marching around like maniacs. I send him a big smile and a subtle wave of my hand, and then the unexpected happens.

"Cadet! Eyes forward, cup your hands, arms in tight!" he screams at the top of his voice.

What is happening? I think to myself. *Oh my goodness.* The others in my E-2 group are now terrified and wondering, *What did this guy do?*

"Yes, sir," I holler in return.

"I'm not a sir. I'm a sergeant. I work for a living," he belts back.

"Yes, Sergeant," I respond and head on my way.

Yikes. Even though it's role playing, it is still daunting. I wonder how Cathy is faring. I let what just happened soak in. Pretty neat to get chewed out by our own cadet. Wink, wink.

The morning hours quickly pass, and before too long, we meet up in Washington Hall for lunch. The other volunteers seated at our table are thrilled to have Nate, a real live-in-person West Point cadet, join them. They toss a few questions his way, and we collectively laugh and smile from the Mock R-Day events that transpired earlier. Our efforts are officially recognized with a certificate of appreciation:

> In recognition of your support during R-Day rehearsal on 28 June 2019. Your selfless assistance and portrayal as a new cadet candidate has greatly enhanced our preparation to receive the West Point Class of 2023. Thanks for a job well done.
>
> Signed: Jason M. Halloran, Colonel, US Army, Acting Commandant of Cadets

The excitement of European travels doesn't end with Nate's return from his AIAD. Sam is up next. One month following Nate's arrival back, we are saying our goodbyes to Sam at Pittsburgh's

International Airport—Pittsburgh to Toronto, Canada to Paris. Sam is traveling with his high school French and Spanish club and chaperones to tour France and Spain. Sam fits right in and captures, perhaps, the most iconic tourist snapshot in Paris, holding and pinching the Eiffel tower in his hand. It's all about depth perception. This classic pose is a must, and Sam perfectly captures the moments and subject. Neat stuff! He provides us with daily text updates on his tourist stops and entertaining critiques of the group's evening dinner cuisine. Maybe he has a future as a food critic. Our seventeen-year-old has taken his first steps into the world of international travel—Toronto, Paris, Bordeaux, Biarittz, Pamplona, and Barcelona. Cathy and I can't help but wonder, *Where will life's journeys take our youngest child?*

In July 2019, Nate sees the next chapter of his West Point adventure highlighted with his assignment to cadet first sergeant for E-2 Company. He's thrilled to be tasked with his newfound responsibilities and even happier to be issued the chevron with the diamond underneath those three-winged sergeant stripes.

I think the news provides a huge confidence boost to Nate as he enters his Cow (third-year cadet) field training. No shortage of training details for the Corps of Cadets as they progress from Plebe to Yearling to Cow and, finally, Firstie status. Nate completes his leadership detail as a squad leader for cadet basic training (a.k.a. Beast) at Camp Buckner, and we gladly welcome him back home for a ten-day break. Nate's return home was uneventful, always a good thing. We can't say the same for Sam's return. Our young man gets to experience firsthand the trials and tribulations of travel, particularly international travel. A delayed return flight departing Madrid to Toronto starts off the trip back home. And when they finally arrive in Toronto, well, a missed connecting flight compounded by dealing with a less-than-customer-friendly travel agency. When the dust settles, Sam and his group end up returning home via a bus ride from Toronto to Buffalo, New York, met with a change of buses, and finally a 1:00 AM arrival in Somerset. Home sweet home!

Both boys are home, safe and sound, in Mom's care. Cathy makes reservations at Prince Gallitzin State Park for a cabin along the lake. Time to get away for a bit, enjoy the outdoors, hike, fish, kayak, and leisurely sit around the campfire. There's something about the smell of wood burning, along with a slight breeze fanning the flames and nonsensical conversation with family on a cool evening in the woods. Relaxing, trancelike, and hypnotic. Love it! But without a doubt, my favorite part of camping is the very first morning. Cathy always lets me sleep in to awake to the smell of bacon sizzling, fresh coffee brewing, orange juice and milk placed on the table, and the pièce de résistance is her triple-berry pancakes—raspberries, blueberries, and blackberries. Delicious!

On the evening before we depart, we decide to see *Toy Story 4* at a nearby drive-in movie theatre. We stop and treat ourselves to ice cream along the way. Then later in the evening, in the pitch-black darkness, while sitting in our picnic chairs next to the car three quarters of the way into the movie, a skunk parades directly in front of us. We hurriedly jump into the car, frantically dashing out of harm's way to avoid getting sprayed. Whew! That ends the night, and we decide to head back to the cabin after that excitement. No matter. Nate wants to wake up at the very crack of dawn and give fishing one last attempt to nab one of these elusive monsters of the lake. He missed a nice one yesterday and is hell-bent on hooking one before throwing in the towel in defeat. Tomorrow is soon here, and Nate and I make our way to the lake, our breath cutting through the cool morning air, where we are walking through the thick mist. Being blanketed in this shroud of fog reminds me of the evening before A-Day when we departed Ike Hall after watching the Tuskegee Airmen show.

Nate casts out into the heavy cloudlike atmosphere of minute water droplets. I hear his yellowish green Reed-Runner spinner lure hit the water in the distance and the click of his bait casting fishing reel. *Bam!*

"Dad!" he excitedly hollers over to me. "I got one on!"

I walk toward him and watch the tip of his rod, bent and bouncing away with a fighter on the other end. This time, Nate is on the winning side. He battles a prize-winning largemouth bass and successfully reels it along the side of the dock where I reach down and pull it out. Two gentlemen are preparing to launch their boat while I'm taking pictures of Nate holding his prized catch.

"I'd wish you good luck," the one gentleman says. "But it looks like you don't need it."

We wish them good luck as well, and after another forty-five minutes or so of fishing, we join Cathy and Sam in the cabin with our fish story and evidence to support it. Today, we have a small black slate tile hanging in our kitchen that reads, FISHERMAN'S CODE: Early to Bed, Early to Rise, Fish like Hell, and Make Up Lies. No lies on this foggy morning.

Another foggy morning greets Nate but this time on the grounds where on July 1–3, 1863, an estimated fifty-one thousand casualties from Union and Confederate forces battled in the bloodiest battle of the Civil War in Gettysburg, Pennsylvania.

The staff leaders of the Corps of Cadets visited Gettysburg for a team-building event in mid-August. All company commanders, first sergeants, and higher-level leaders made the trip. As the first-semester chain of command, the cadet leaders had the opportunity to reflect and team build through a close examination of leadership, valor, and decision-making of the Battle of Gettysburg. Many of the USMA senior leaders addressed the cadets throughout the week, providing a wealth of knowledge and experience that solidified the lessons learned on the battlefield.

Nate gets a surprise visit from Hillary when she steps away from her motherly duties and meets up with him at his hotel on his final evening. With ice-cream cones in hand, Hillary sends a picture of the two of them and catches Cathy and I off guard. Such a joy seeing brother and sister together, huge smiles, and Hillary encouraging Nate, showing her excitement with Nate's first sergeant assignment.

Nate, back at West Point on August 18, along with the other cadets of the Class of 2021, affirmed their commitment to service in the US Army during a ceremony where they dressed in their India white uniforms. This is truly the point of no return without being tagged with financial or military service consequences. Nate and his classmates take the Oath of Affirmation, binding them to complete their next two years of study and a minimum of five years of active-duty service thereafter. Joining the affirmation ceremony were members of the West Point Class of 1971, the fifty-year affiliation class for the Class of 2021, who presented the cadets with commemorative coins to mark the occasion.

Hard to believe our not-so-long ago Plebe is now a Cow. These forty-seven months are flying by! And before we know it, we are once again seated in Lincoln-Financial Field, our third Army versus Navy game. This time, however, our cadet has his name announced during the pregame march on, in front of thousands of spectators and many more on national television. We proudly stand, beaming, as the stadium echoes with the words from the broadcast announcer, "Company E is commanded by Cadet Captain Robert Anderson of Greenwich, Connecticut. The first sergeant is Cadet First Sergeant Nathaniel Olsavsky from Friedens, Pennsylvania."

Taking in the enormity of the activities before us, watching both midshipmen and cadets alike marching on, all I can think is, *God bless these young men and women.*

It would have taken divine intervention on this cold, rainy December 14 day to save Army as the Black Knights are outplayed and outmatched by a much-tougher Navy team, 31–7, keeping our fingers crossed for the next match up in 2020. Congratulations, Navy! The Commander in Chief's Trophy is yours.

Things quickly turn for the better as the fall semester comes to an end. On top of that, the Eisenhower Barracks' renovation is complete and those cadets housed in Bradley Barracks will have a new home, new accommodations with air-conditioning and the sort, when they return in January to start the spring semester. And the message comes down that Cows who were first sergeants will be permitted to bring a personal vehicle back to West Point rather than waiting until the end of spring break. Nate, along with thirty-four others, are thrilled! He has his eyes set on taking the Jeep Cherokee back to West Point. Now, yep now, Cathy and I need to figure out the best way to break the news to Sam. The Jeep has been all his with Nate away.

Being part of the leadership detail comes with all kinds of responsibilities. Before Nate can leave for Christmas break, he's tasked with overseeing that the storage rooms in Bradley Barracks are moved to Ike and properly cleaned out. He's picked up some interesting vernacular, much like Uncle Tommy. He's not a happy camper. But the duty comes with a perk. He comes across an unclaimed, unaccounted-for Fender Squier Classic Vibe '60s Telecaster Thinline Electric guitar in a black guitar case. From the dust and aged, slightly rust-covered bridge, and tainted pickup screws, it is obvious the guitar has been in storage for some time. Nate puts out an all-points bulletin in an attempt to find the owner, but to no avail.

Being a guitar player himself, his chain of command gives him the go-ahead to take it. An early Christmas present perhaps. My coworker plays, builds, and repairs guitars and gives the fretboard a thorough cleaning, replaces the strings, and polishes the entire body and other parts. It looks amazing and sounds great!

Cathy and I get our own form of an early Christmas gift as well—a letter from one of Nate's instructors in the Department of Civil and Mechanical Engineering arrives in the mail:

> *Dear Mr. and Mrs. Olsavsky,*
> *It is with profound pride that I am writing to inform you of Nathaniel's achievement in my course, Thermal-Fluid Systems I (MC311)… Achieving an A+ in MC311 is no small feat as most cadets who take the class identify it as the "most difficult class at West Point." The fact that he excelled while balancing competing responsibilities as a Company First Sergeant makes this feat even more impressive… I look forward to witnessing his progress throughout his remaining time at the Academy and during his Army career. You should be very proud of him!*

Yes, we are proud. We are thankful and we are ecstatic for Nate, for our strong, healthy, and happy grandson, and for Sam who is fully recovered. Nate is excelling; we are blessed.

Hard to believe Christmas 2019 has arrived. By this time next year, Nate will have received his Army branch assignment; this is where he'll start his career upon graduation. West Point and the Army just implemented a new process to assign branches called the

Market Modeling Branching System. The new model pairs cadets with a branch by considering how they rank the seventeen branches, but now the commandants of each branch also have a vote in which cadets receive their branch assignment. Nate's top choices are Corps of Engineers, Air Defense Artillery, and Signal Corps. Next Christmas will certainly be different; we'll be checking out what Army branch insignia Nate will be wearing. What won't be different, however, is Cathy's holiday meal preparation—baked honey glazed ham, home-made horseradish, kielbasa, halupki (stuffed cabbage), potato salad, deviled eggs, buttered rolls, pickled beets and eggs, green bean casserole, and a cookie tray that serves as a grab-and-go snack throughout the day. Diets are put aside over the holidays!

Everyone successfully made their way onto Santa's nice list as colorful gift-wrapped packages of all shapes and sizes are under the brightly lit ornate spruce tree. Sam, Nate, Hillary and Jacob, and Cody are all smiles. Cathy and I helped Santa's elves with one of Nate's gifts this year, one that shows a personal connection to the past—a shadow box. We assembled a collection of World War I items of Nate's great-grandfather and had the ensemble professionally framed at Michael's, an arts and crafts chain store. A twenty-nine-by-twenty-seven-inch brown, gold-lipped distressed frame with sage wood backing to mount the *Pointer View* article commemorating the one hundredth anniversary of WWI. We match the article with my grandfather Joseph Liko's Army discharge papers, a photograph of both him and my grandmother, Rose Elias Liko, along with a picture of Camp Gordon, Georgia, the location where he was discharged.

The framer at Michael's does an outstanding job center-ing the items and laying out the design for the remaining items: a WWI Victory Medal with the words *The Great War for Civilization 1914–1919*, an enlisted Army hat badge and US pin, Army private stripes, Eighty-Second Airborne patch, and challenge coins com-memorating the one-hundredth-year anniversary of the Eighty-Second Airborne Division and the end of the First World War.

I imagine that, one day, Nate will hang the shadow box in his home office, along with the many other Army career memorabilia items he'll have gathered over the years.

And speaking of years, we welcome in yet another new year. Happy 2020! The holiday break comes to an end and Nate makes his solo trip back to West Point. Not as a passenger on a bus, but rather him and the Jeep Cherokee. Nate is thrilled that we gave him the green light to take the car back to West Point. And Sam? His spirits pick up when my job goes to a fully remote home-based position. This frees up a vehicle, and once again, he's able to drive to school on his own. Nothing like keeping both boys happy.

February turns out to be a busy month for us. We make a trip to Daytona, Florida, to visit Embry-Riddle Aeronautical University. Sam is planning to dual major in aerospace and mechanical engineering upon graduation and has narrowed his choices between Embry-Riddle and West Virginia University (WVU). After our WVU engineering orientation visit at the end of the month, it's final; Sam makes his decision. Let's go, WVU Mountaineers! We're so thrilled for him, and his senior year is flying by and coming down the homestretch. Cathy and I will be empty nesters soon enough, with the exception of Cody.

A key milestone in every college student's life is their twenty-first birthday. And Nate is no exception. "Happy birthday, Nate!" We wish him from afar. He's been taken under the wings of his cadet brothers and sisters and celebrates at the West Point Firstie Club. Cheers! A draft beer in his hand, leaning in for a sip sends Cathy into an emotional spin, and I see the tears building in her eyes as she repeatedly looks at the pic. Some things never change for a mom. Not sad tears but teardrops of passage. Another big step for her and for our son.

The excitement continues in Nate's small corner of the world. On February 10, he selects his Class of 2021 cadet ring. Over the Christmas holiday break, Nate showed us the United States Military Academy, West Point Official 2021 Ring Catalog by Balfour. Such a cool thing to share this experience with Nate. He and Cathy go through the ring styles, options, finish, divider stones, and top stone options. Only as a mother and son could do; the mother-son bond is unbreakable, impenetrable, and cast purely in none other than love, just like the look from Cathy seeing Sam in the hospital ICU room and the look at seeing Hillary and Noah together. It continues with Cody; with Cathy sitting in her chair, he jumps next to her and lays his chin across her lap and lets out a deep sigh. Yeah, he has a favorite, a mother's love without a doubt.

The stone selection for Nate's class ring is his and his alone. And we are in complete agreement with his pick—peridot. Peridot is one of the few gemstones that occur in only one color: an olive green. A perfect match for Army and West Point and his future *pinks and greens*. The United States Army is changing their service uniform. The new look? It chose a uniform that looks like the old green gabardine wool field coat and khaki trousers that officers wore in World War II. The troops who beat the Axis powers in the 1940s gave the service uniform, with its slightly rose-hued trousers or skirt and distinctive belted olive coat, an affectionate nickname: pinks and greens.

We can't wait until he begins his Firstie year, a cadet wearing the red sash, then to celebrate the Class of 2021 Ring Ceremony with him in August.

But shortly after he comes home for spring 2020, breaking news on when a return trip back to West Point becomes uncertain and up in the air.

Shock waves and a whirlwind of uncertainty ripple worldwide when on March 11, 2020, the World Health Organization declares a global pandemic due to the outbreak of the novel coronavirus, COVID-19. On March 13, 2020, a national emergency was declared in the United States concerning the COVID-19 outbreak.

All 24-7 news coverage pummels us. School closures, restaurants shuttered, church services cancelled, travel locked down, and toilet paper shortages. On March 19, 2020, Lt. Gen. Darryl A. Williams, superintendent of the United States Military Academy, announced that the Corps of Cadets would not be returning from spring break as planned. Our cadet is home to stay until we hear otherwise.

As so often happens, when one door closes, another opens. Such is the case with our family. In the midst of the adversity before the world, our family finds resiliency that helps us deal with these crazy times. Stumbling blocks turn into small wonderful gifts before our very eyes.

Daily walks with Cody become a mainstay. Early-spring trout fishing drives Nate and me outdoors—in the sun, heavy downpours, and even a late-spring snow shower, 30°F. Go figure. But the fish are biting and catching a mix of brook, brown, and rainbow trout are etched in our memories. Up next is an all-out, hands-on-deck family project to construct a stone patio and firepit adjacent to our deck. Dixie pink stone gravel provides the base and an ornamental stone border finish off the design. Nate completes his spring semester online followed by two additional courses while remaining at home. We have the pleasure to celebrate, in the comfort of our living room, Nate's induction into two academic honor societies: Phi Kappa Phi, the oldest and most exclusive honor society in the country, and Tau Beta Pi, the oldest engineering honor society. Locally, Nate and three Naval Academy students are the subject of a news article in our hometown newspaper—"Service academy students adapting to studying at home."

Our highlight is having Nate home to join us, as a complete family, to celebrate Sam's high school graduation. Hillary and Nate share in Sam's excitement. Sam was so worried that Nate wouldn't be able to see him graduate given Nate's summer training schedule. But as it turned out, that brother-brother bond was further solidified. A visit to see the WVU campus, Sam's next new stomping grounds where he plans to double-major in aerospace & mechanical engineering, was the icing on the cake.

What comes to mind? "There's no other love like the love for a brother. There's no other love like the love from a brother." Those words take us back over three years ago to that bright, sunny July 2, 2017, morning departure from our home to West Point. Excitement, fear, and a journey into the unknown. Now an early 5:00 am Sunday, July 26, 2020, morning departure and there remain many unknowns. A return trip back to West Point, not as a Plebe rather as a Firstie— the Cadet in the Red Sash. We say our goodbyes. We wipe our tears. We give our son a final hug and kiss.

"We love you, Nate." Quietly, Cody rolls over, yes, as if to say, "Nate, I love you! Be safe and see you soon."

CHAPTER 8

A Compilation of the Volumes: *The Adventures of Cadet Cody* Highlights

THANK YOU FOR joining us along our West Point journey as we revisited the tales and exploits of our emotional passage from R-Day, Beast, March Back, Acceptance Day, the December 8, 2017, Army-Navy win, Plebe Parent Weekend, and Sabalauski Air Assault School!

It's been an evolving, exhilarating, and astonishing ride. We wouldn't have it any other way! Make no mistake, we've had our ups and downs along the way. Like so many story bylines, we laughed, we cried. Most importantly, we stayed strong. We have been so very blessed. New faces, new friends, incredible experiences.

Nate has visited the US Air Force Academy in Colorado Springs, Colorado, and the US Coast Guard Academy in New London, Connecticut. He has listened to Medal of Honor recipients share their harrowing stories of sacrifice. He has sat before and listened to President George W. Bush and the Honorable Leon E. Panetta speak as Sylvanus Thayer Award Recipients. Nate has been fortunate to hear one of our favorite TV actors, Alan Alda, otherwise known as Captain Hawkeye Pierce from the *M*A*S*H* TV series, lecture to the cadets. And as a surprise birthday gift, he gave me a signed copy of Alan Alda's book, *If I Understood You, Would I Have This Look* *on My Face? My Adventures in the Art and Science of Relating and Communicating.*

Funny how things work. The gift of one book creates momentum for the creation of another.

Plebe year at West Point has provided our family with not just twelve months but also a lifetime of incredible memories. One in particular that stands out was pinning Nate with the National Defense Service Medal (NDSM) during Plebe Parent Weekend. His first medal! Some background for you. The NDSM is a decoration presented to recognize all military members who have served in active duty during a declared *national emergency*. To be eligible, members must have served honorably during one of the following time periods: the Korean War from June 27, 1950–July 27, 1954; the Vietnam War from January 1, 1961–August 14, 1974; the Gulf War from August 2, 1990–November 30, 1995; the War on Terrorism from September 11, 2001 and a yet-to-be-determined date.

West Point cadets are considered eligible according to Army Regulation 600–8–22 Ch. 2–10.f. Cadets of the US Military Academy are eligible for the NDSM, during any of the inclusive periods listed above, upon completion of the oath swearing-in ceremonies as a cadet.

On this evening, many of the cadet companies gathered in the Central Area. Parents and family members alike met our cadets. E-2's TAC officer assembled the cadets and read the announcement for awarding the NDSM. Similar companies were in the midst of the same thing.

Then family members and friends were called forward to pin their cadets. I stepped forward, removed the medal from its case, and pinned it squarely on Nate's dress gray uniform. And once again, I was wiping tears from my eyes, quietly following with a firm hug of my son. Such a proud feeling!

I was fortunate to also pin one of his fellow E-2 company members whose family couldn't make it to Plebe Parent Weekend. It was an honor, and I will always remember that celebrated cold evening and those crisp, clear, and standout moments.

It is our hope that *The Adventures of Cadet Cody* series highlights does justice to these memories. We auspiciously completed eleven volumes in the Cadet Cody memoirs over the course of Nate's Plebe year at West Point. To no surprise, three of these Cadet Cody story lines found their way to Nate during his six weeks of cadet basic training in the hot and humid weeks of July and August 2017. The others were a continuing saga capturing and reflecting our cadet's real time Plebe activities. All-night guard duty, PT, marching, the House of Tears, and hand grenades—all part of the foundation leading up to the beginnings of Army life and a future US Army second lieutenant.

More often than not, we tied these events into the Cadet Cody adventure title. For example, volume 9, March 27, 2018, is titled "Plebe Parent Weekend! And Now Boxing" Easy enough to see what our theme is focused on.

The cast of characters, locations, and story ideas in the Cadet Cody series were plentiful. The star, of course, is our beloved dog, Cody. Also featured are his canine cousins, Stella and Remi. These two playful dogs are our daughter Hillary and son-in-law Jacob's blue and red Australian cattle dogs. The running joke in our family is that Stella is Cody's girlfriend. A lot of background behind this relationship. Even after having Cody neutered and Stella spayed, Cody never fails to chase and attempt to mount Stella.

Yikes! Enough said!

Cathy, our teenage son, Sam, and I make numerous appearances in *The Adventures of Cadet Cody* editions, as do Hillary and Jacob. Coming in as best supporting actor, not surprisingly, is our USMA West Point cadet, Nate.

Our backyard in Friedens, Pennsylvania, provides a recurring backdrop for many of the photo ops. A beach vacation, hike at a nearby state park, and Nate's friend also make for adventurous and heartwarming storyboard callouts.

So there you have it! That is some of the background on these cartoonlike stories. Without further ado, here are the eleven *Adventures in Cadet Cody* volume titles. Take a moment to soak up the relatable themes. I guarantee you will walk away with a handful of smiles and perhaps a few chuckles.

So don't delay. *Adventures of Cadet Cody: The True Story of How One Family (and Their Pet Dog) Survived R-Day, Beast, and Plebe Year at West Point* volumes await you!

Listing of Cadet Cody volumes:

Volume 1: "The Adventures of Cadet Cody," July 24, 2017

Volume 2: "The Early Years," July 31, 2017

Volume 3: "Camp Barkner," August 9, 2017

Volume 4: "From New Cadet to Plebe, Making Cadets Great Again," September 6, 2017

Volume 5: "Family Weekend at USMA West Point," October 17, 2017

Volume 6: "The Buildup to Army Versus Navy," November 29, 2017

Volume 7: "Merry Christmas from the Corps of Cadets," December 25, 2017

Volume 8: "Christmas 2017 Was Great! But Where Is Spring—Brrrr?" January 18, 2018

Volume 9: "Plebe Parent Weekend! And Now Boxing" March 27, 2018

Volume 10: "Up Next Is Sabalauski Air Assault School," May 31, 2018

Volume 11: "I'm a Yearling Now and Look What I Can Do," August 22, 2018

Volume 1: The Adventures of Cadet Cody, July 24, 2017

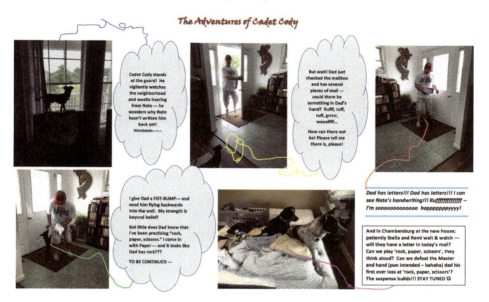

What the Story Is About

The first volume of Cadet Cody came about as a simple way to send Nate pictures while he was at CBT. Cathy was looking at Cody, standing tall on his favorite chair, looking out into the front yard. Click, there's a pic. Out of the blue, she named him Cadet Cody. The name stuck. I'm not exactly sure how Cathy and I got on the subject, but we started talking about a story with Cadet Cody. Hmm, I thought. Let's do a cartoon! *The Adventures of Cadet Cody* was born.

At this time, mid-July 2017, we were still anxiously awaiting our first letter from our cadet. A few more pics emerged. And then it came! Nate's first letter! An adrenaline rush!

As far as the rock paper scissors call out, well, I have the claim to fame in our family of never having lost a rock paper scissors match! Although I've been accused of, uh-huh...of all things, cheating. Unfounded accusations, I say! I maintain my record is a solid 1,783 wins, 0 losses, 1 tie. One tie! Of all things, 1 tie that blemishes my perfect record. To this day, one disputed match with Hillary when she was six years old! Go figure. And the family stories of the rock paper scissors disputes are for another time.

What We Really Liked about This Volume

This was our inaugural launch. It tapped into everything. Cody, Stella, and Remi were easy targets. Anything and everything was in play when it came to sharing pics on our iPhones. And it became a nice way to deal with the no-contact reality. The callouts stretched and challenged our imaginations, and we knew Nate would get a kick out of seeing what we were up to.

Did You Know?

West Point was the first American university to adopt class rings. The only two classes not to have class rings were 1836 (opted to have no rings) and 1879 (chose to have class cufflinks).

Also, the US Military Academy's coat of arms displays the Greek symbols of wisdom and military virtue, the helmet and sword of Pallas Athene upon the American shield. "Duty, honor, country" is the academy's motto. This was adopted as the academy coat of arms on 8 October 1898.

Volume 2: The Early Years, July 31, 2017

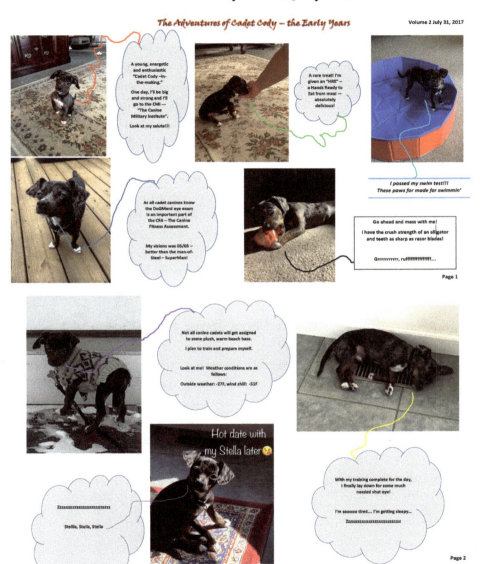

What the Story Is About

We were writing Nate letters about all our day-to-day happenings, with letters going out at least every other day. Family cookouts, local weather, what we had for dinner if we went out for an evening, and something as simple as cutting the grass. And we also had a few short letters in our hands from Nate as well—*finally*, contact with our cadet. Things appeared to be going well at Beast. The House of Tears, rifle qualification, PT, marching and drilling, academic testing—all falling into place.

The pics of Cody in this volume touched upon Nate's entire West Point journey from SLE through the nomination process and ending with an appointment in hand. Nate got some good laughs out of Cody's physical fitness and his grit and fortitude: swim test, CFA, and Cody's choice of post/base assignment. And then there's always Stella. She's always on his mind. Sounds like a Willy Nelson song, doesn't it?

What We Really Liked about This Volume

The picture on our deck of Cody squinting is priceless and tied nicely with the steps for admission to the USMA. Then, they have to be medically qualified. An easy play on words and we turned the Department of Defense Medical Examination Review Board (DoDMERB) into DoGMERD. All part of the canine fitness assessment (CFA) or, more appropriately, the candidate fitness assessment.

A strong performance on the CFA is an absolute must to get an appointment into West Point, whether you are dog or human!

Did You Know?

The West Point Class of 1915 would become known as the class the stars fell on. Of 164 men who graduated, 59 achieved the rank of brigadier general or higher.

Two five-star generals and two four-star generals, seven three-star lieutenant generals, twenty-four two-star major generals, and twenty-four one-star brigadier generals.

Among the most notable names were US President and Supreme Allied Commander Dwight D. Eisenhower and first Chairman of the Joint Chiefs of Staff Omar Bradley.

The story of these unique and historic men from the graduating Class of 1915 is detailed in the book written by Michael E. Haskew, *West Point 1915: Eisenhower, Bradley, and the Class the Stars Fell On.*

Volume 3: Camp Barkner, August 9, 2017

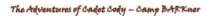

The Adventures of Cadet Cody — Camp BARKner   Volume 3 August 9, 2017

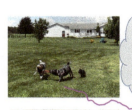

Cadet Cody, Stella and Remi enjoy some down time and playful action before making the march out to Camp Barkner.

"We're ready!"

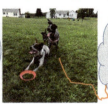

None too soon!!!

The order is given—

"... get in line, gear ready...

and MARCH you Canines!"

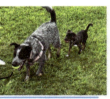

LEFT, RIGHT, LEFT! Stay in tight Cadets! Now sing you pile of fur and teeth!

Mama Mama can't you see,
what the Army's done to me.
They put me in a barber's chair,
spun me around I have no hair.
Mama Mama can't you see,
what the army's done to me.
They took away my favorite jeans,
now I'm wearing Army greens.

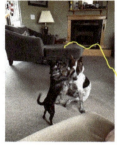

Boxing is mandatory at The Academy.

And yes, the Cadets jump right into training!

Cadet Cody takes on one of the star Frisbee athletes — Remi.

...Cadet Cody goes in for the knockout punch!!!

KA-POW!

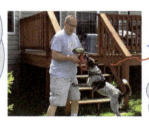

Here....Remi is on his first shift of afternoon guard duty at Camp Barkner.

"He's ready!" Attack mode kicks in as he tackles an intruder!

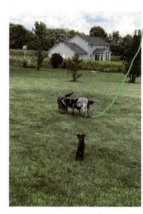

Cadet Cody leads his Squad in maneuvers.

— He checks on their readiness.

YES SIR!

These Canine Cadets are looking **EXCEPTIONAL!**

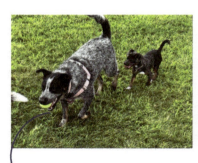

In the meantime, more drilling and marching...LEFT, RIGHT, LEFT! NOW SOUND OFF!

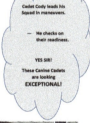

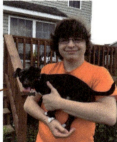

"Oh, those were the days"

"Sam would carry me and scratch my belly and rub my shoulders."

They say that in the Army, the pay is mighty fine
They give you a 100 dollars and take back 99.
They say that in the Army, the coffee's mighty fine
It looks like muddy water, and tastes like turpentine.
They say that in the Army, the biscuits are mighty fine
One rolled off the table and killed a friend of mine.
They say that in the Army, the meat is mighty fine
Last night we had ten puppies, this morning only nine.

What the Story Is About

Stella, Remi, and Cody found their way out to our backyard many times during that early August 2017 weekend. We were dog sitting for Hillary and Jacob while they took a much-needed break from the many hours of hard work as new homeowners. The pups, as we often referred to the three amigo canines, loved to chase the frisbee and fetch tennis balls. Pictures of their shenanigans quickly found their way onto our iPhone camera albums.

August 19, 2017, Acceptance Day (A-Day), was getting closer and closer.

What We Really Liked about This Volume

To this day, Nate still chuckles about Camp Barkner, along with CBT, or canine basic training. Love it! Cody's knockout punch on Remi is a favorite too.

And Sam's hair is unmistakably out of control. I should be so lucky to have a full head of hair.

Most importantly, we were in countdown mode to A-Day. To say we were anxious is an understatement.

Did You Know?

A 1973 episode of the famed TV series *M*A*S*H* referenced a fictional Army-Navy football game that ended 42–36 Navy. To this day, no Army-Navy game has ended with that score. The radio announcer in the episode says the game is the Fifty-Third Army-Navy game. That game was actually played in 1952. Navy won, 7–0.

Volume 4: From New Cadet to Plebe, Making Cadets Great Again, September 6, 2017

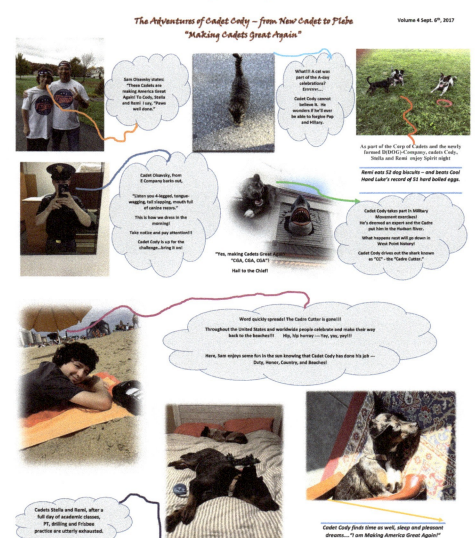

The Adventures of Cadet Cody – from New Cadet to Plebe
"Making Cadets Great Again"

Volume 4 Sept. 6th, 2017

Sam Olsavsky states: "These Cadets are making America Great Again! To Cody, Stella and Remi I say, "Paws well done."

What!!! A cat was part of the A-day celebrations? Errrrrrrr....

Cadet Cody cannot believe it. He wonders if he'll ever be able to forgive Pap and Hillary.

As part of the Corp of Cadets and the newly formed D(DOG)-Company, cadets Cody, Stella and Remi enjoy Spirit night

Cadet Olsavsky, from E Company barks out,

"Listen you 4-legged, tongue-wagging, tail slapping, mouth full of canine razors."

This is how we dress in the morning!

Take notice and pay attention!!!

Cadet Cody is up for the challenge...bring it on!

Remi eats 52 dog biscuits – and beats Cool Hand Luke's record of 51 hard boiled eggs.

Cadet Cody takes part in Military Movement exercises! He's deemed an expert and the Cadre put him in the Hudson River.

What happens next will go down in West Point history!

Cadet Cody drives out the shark known as "CC" - the "Cadre Cutter."

"Yes, making Cadets Great Again" "CGA, CGA, CGA"!

Hail to the Chief!

Word quickly spreads! The Cadre Cutter is gone!!!

Throughout the United States and worldwide people celebrate and make their way back to the beaches!!! Hip, hip hurray ---Yay, yay, yay!!!

Here, Sam enjoys some fun in the sun knowing that Cadet Cody has done his job — Duty, Honor, Country, and Beaches!

Cadets Stella and Remi, after a full day of academic classes, PT, drilling and Frisbee practice are utterly exhausted.

Cadet Cody finds time as well, sleep and pleasant dreams...."I am Making America Great Again!"

Page 2

What the Story Is About

Nate is now officially a Plebe. A-Day was an incredible experience. We rented a house in Cornwall-on-the-Hudson and had our first opportunity to spend time with Nate. A neighborhood feline was a constant visitor on the front porch, keeping Pap company as he made his way outside to the fresh rising activities near the riverside to enjoy his early-morning cup of coffee. I'm sure Cody would have been beside himself throwing a fit if we had brought him along.

That following weekend, Cathy, Sam, Hillary, and I made our way to Ocean City, Maryland, for some beach-side fun in the sun. Summer vacation was quickly dwindling from weeks to days, but we made the most of it. Two visits to West Point, March Back, and A-Day, then to Ocean City, Maryland, for some sun, sand, surf, and seafood dining.

What We Really Liked about This Volume

Sam and I attended then candidate Trump's presidential rally in Johnstown, Pennsylvania, on October 22, 2016. The pic of Sam and I worked well for our Making Cadets Great Again theme. And the D (Dog) Company scene with our oh so familiar canine threesome stars is a keeper.

We took in the Ocean City, Maryland, boardwalk and came upon a building with a great white shark bursting through the upper floor. This shark now goes by the name of the cadre cutter!

We are now getting more adept and skilled with our writing and creativity expanding additional volumes in *The Adventure of Cadet Cody* series.

But most important of all, we know these stories provide a touch of home and an inspirational burst of love and energy for Nate.

Did You Know?

Sedgwick's Spurs, a monument to Civil War Union General John Sedgwick stands on the outskirts of the Plain. Sedgwick's bronze statue has spurs with rowels that freely rotate. Legend states that if a cadet is in danger of failing a class, they are to don their full-dress parade uniform the night before the final exam. The cadet visits the statue and spins the rowels at the stroke of midnight. Then the cadet runs back to their barracks as fast as he or she can. According to legend, if Sedgwick's ghost catches them, they will fail the exam. Otherwise, the cadet will pass the exam and the course. Although being out of their rooms after midnight is officially against regulations, violations have been known to be overlooked for the sake of tradition.

Volume 5: Family Weekend at USMA
West Point, October 17, 2017

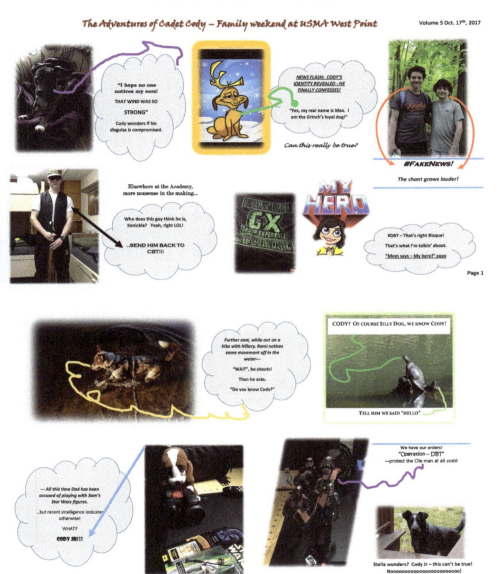

What the Story Is About

This was our first experience with Family Weekend at West Point. Our first Army football game too against Temple and a win! Nate sent us a pic of him dressed up for their usual Thursday Spirit Dinner. Sporting sunglasses and a slicked-back look, he was stylin'. This provided us with an opportunity to resurrect his role as Kinickie from his high school performance in *Grease*.

The "do you know Cody?" question is a family favorite. Anytime we pass someone walking their dog or other pet or see a deer, raccoon, opossum, rabbit, wild turkey, etc., we jokingly belt out this question.

Hillary and Jacob were enjoying their time with Stella and Remi at a Pennsylvania state park lake so the picture of Remi worked in nicely along with the basking turtles. Lastly, we have a stuffed animal twin of Cody, whom we conveniently named Cody Jr. Sam's assorted collection of Star Wars figures was a constant target of being *mysteriously* moved from their positions time to time. Of course, yours truly would be accused, wrongly perhaps, of the alleged crime. But as you can clearly see, this story reveals the true culprit. It was Cody Jr. all along!

What We Really Liked about This Volume

Cody's pic of his ears in the wind lay the foundation for his secret identity—Max, the Grinch's loyal dog. Throwback memories and reminiscing about Nate's role in *Grease* brought warmth to our hearts of those bygone days. And Hillary's pictures of the turtles soaking up the sun on a stump in the lake was perfect!

Did You Know?

The US Civil War had a total of 294 graduates from West Point serving as officers for the Union. The Confederacy had a total of 151 of its officers that were graduates of the US Military Academy. During the war, there were 60 major battles. In every one of these, there was at least one USMA graduate commanding one side or the other or both.

Volume 6: The Buildup to Army Versus Navy, November 29, 2017

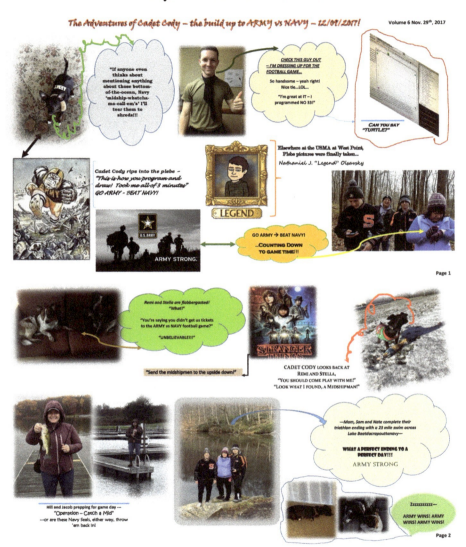

What the Story Is About

This is all about Army versus Navy and Thanksgiving too! Nate made his way home for Thanksgiving by way of his roommate. So convenient for us. One less trip back and forth. And the hot topic being discussed on the social media pages was Plebe pictures.

That November 2017 weekend was cold and chilly, but nonetheless, we planned an early-morning hike at nearby Laurel Hill State Park. It was relaxing, and we could just feel it in the air that winter's grip was racing at a fast pace right around the corner.

What We Really Liked about This Volume

Hillary and Jacob are avid bass fisherman. And on one of those late autumn weekends, Hill outfished her hubby. Nice catch, Hill!

This volume also contains a lot of playful banter with Navy. The picture of Nate, Sam, and Cathy on our hike made for the perfect play on words with Lake Beatdacrapouttanavy in the backdrop. Go, Army! Beat Navy!

Did You Know?

Boxing and combative at West Point are the only mandatory activities that pits one cadet against another in full-body contact. It teaches fear management, which is a necessary skill to lead soldiers in combat. Cadets are closely monitored and the program objectives are driven by a safety-first environment.

West Point made the historic decision to integrate the boxing requirement in the summer of 2016 that now includes both women and men.

Volume 7: Merry Christmas from the Corps of Cadets, December 25, 2017

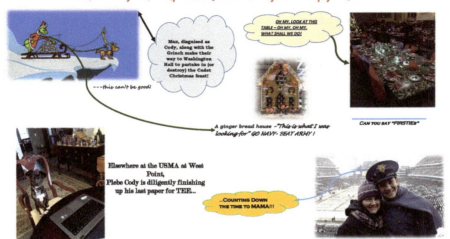

The Adventures of Cadet Cody – MERRY CHRISTMAS from the Corp of Cadets! Volume 7 Dec. 25th, 2017

Max, disguised as Cody, along with the Grinch make their way to Washington Hall to partake in (or destroy) the Cadet Christmas feast!

---this can't be good!

OH MY, LOOK AT THIS TABLE – OH MY, OH MY, WHAT SHALL WE DO!

A ginger bread house -"This is what I was looking for" GO NAVY- BEAT ARMY !

CAN YOU SAY "FIRSTIES"

Elsewhere at the USMA at West Point, Plebe Cody is diligently finishing up his last paper for TEE...

...COUNTING DOWN THE TIME TO MAMA!!!

Page 1

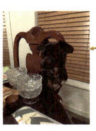

CADET CODY LOOKS AT REMI AND STELLA, "C'MON – LET'S HAVE ANOTHER DRINK!" WE BEAT NAVY 14-13! LET'S KEEP CELEBRATING!!!

"Send the midshipmen back to Annapolis!"

... but Cadet Cody and Cadet Olsavsky's Christmas spirit begin to grow, and along with the Grinch they begin to sing and their hearts are a glow---

"And the Grinch, with his Grinch-feet ice cold in the snow, stood puzzling and puzzling, how could it be so? It came without ribbons. It came without tags. It came without packages, boxes or bags. And he puzzled and puzzled 'till his puzzler was sore. Then the Grinch thought of something he hadn't before. What if Christmas, he thought, doesn't come from a store. What if Christmas, perhaps, means a little bit more. **AND ACTUALLY COMES FROM THE WEST POINT CORP.** **ARMY STRONG**

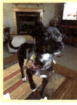

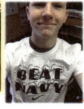

From me and Cadet Olsavsky - Merry Christmas NAVY... And Happy New Year!

Page 2

What the Story Is About

'Tis the season. Army beats Navy 14–13 in an amazing down-to-the-final seconds' finish. A missed field goal by Navy's kicker sealed it! What an incredible experience for our very first Army-Navy football game.

Nate was keeping us up-to-date on the upcoming Christmas dinner and the status of his term end exams (TEEs). Nate and his other Plebe friends made the news on the West Point Instagram page for one of the best Christmas-decorated dinner tables in Washington Hall.

During an early-morning work-from-home day for me, Cody was making himself quite comfortable in front of my laptop. And he tried his best to indulge in some holiday cheer. In the meantime, we were counting down the days until Christmas break.

What We Really Liked about This Volume

Cody shows his true self as Max, the Grinch's right-hand helper. The picture of Nate with his arm around Cathy is heartwarming, and their smiles need no explanation. Finally, in the very truest spirit of the Christmas season, and a few changes in the words of the great Dr. Seuss, Nate wishes Navy a Merry Christmas and Happy New Year! This college football season-ending football game is the *only* game where everyone on the field and from each opposing side (the collective and selfless masses from both the Army and Navy academies) is willing to sacrifice their lives and die for everyone watching this spirited game.

Did You Know?

The tradition of mules as mascots for Army dates back to 1899 when an officer at the Philadelphia Quartermaster Depot decided that the Army team needed a mascot to counter the Navy goat.

Volume 8: Christmas 2017 Was Great! But Where Is Spring—Brrrr? January 18, 2018

The Adventures of Cadet Cody – Christmas 2017 was Great! But where is Spring ---Brrrrrr? Volume 8 January 18th, 2018

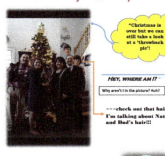

"Christmas is over but we can still take a look at a 'throwback pic'!

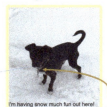

I'm having snow much fun out here!

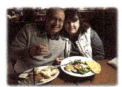

HEY, WHERE AM I?

Why aren't I in the picture? Huh?

---check out that hair! I'm talking about Nate and Dad's hair!!!

...BUT NOT AS MUCH FUN AS MOM AND DAD ARE HAVING!

I WONDER WHAT'S GOING ON OUT ON THE PLAIN AT WEST POINT!!!

"If you think I'm getting out of bed to read announcements, clean up for AMI and drill & do laundry—FORGET IT. " Pure nonsense when the Cadre schedule TAPS for 1:30AM.

Plebe Cody is clearly setting himself up for hours ----and he B-A-R-K-S, "Go ask pretty boy Olsavsky to do all that and see what happens"

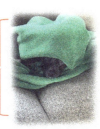

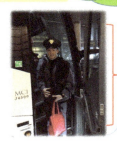

CADET OLSAVSKY IS FULL OF EXCITEMENT AND ANTICIPATION: "MAN, I CAN'T WAIT TO GET BACK FOR ANNOUNCEMENTS & AMI AND SAMI AND DRILL & SOCCER PRACTICE!

...LOVIN' THE PLEBE YEAR – DEAN'S LIST!!!

Page 1

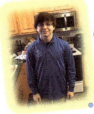

Check out Sam --- he's a workin' Man --- "put your $ in the bank and take your broke home" Who needs the Army

HEY, WE DON'T WANT TO GO OUTSIDE IN THE SNOW! CADET CODY IS ALL BUNDLED UP AND WARM...

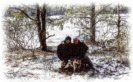

AS SPONGE BOB WOULD SAY..."3 HOURS LATER" Or, as the French state --- « trois heures plus tard »

REMI AND STELLA TRAIN LIKE TRUE SOLDIERS – GO 10TH MOUNTAIN DIVISION!

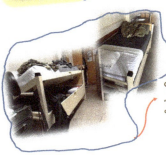

Cadet Olsavsky is quoted in The West Pointer saying: "What was all the fuss with changing rooms? My bed is looking GUDA!"

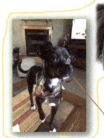

Cadet Cody eyes & zeros in on the elusive Cadet Parka ----oh joy and Sweet Baby Jesus. Wait ------

"They forgot my BrewDog patch!"

Page 2

What the Story Is About

The 2017 holiday season is now in the rearview mirror and a memory. The Western Pennsylvania Parents Club coordinated a charter bus for the return back to West Point for area cadets. This is a huge convenience for parents and saves a roundtrip drive to get Nate back to the academy. So nice!

Sam started working at Hidden Valley Ski Resort and clearly loves getting a paycheck, along with the other perks—*free season ski pass*!

Once again, Stella and Remi make an appearance while hiking and give an appreciative shout-out to the US Army light infantry Tenth Mountain Division based at Fort Drum, New York.

Usually, Nate will let us know when he receives his next-in-line issued new uniform or other clothing, like T-shirts, sweatshirts, etc. We had been hounding him to send a picture of his winter parka, and finally, behold! He is now in the colder, wind-swept, darker days of the winter season and the long gray blanket of what January holds in store for the Hudson Valley.

What We Really Liked about This Volume

Nate made the dean's list in the first semester at West Point! We were so excited and proud, to say the least. He was keeping us up-to-date on his activities too—boxing, IOCT (indoor obstacle course test), APFT, etc. He was glad to be changing rooms because his first semester bunk had a broken latch, with no near-term fix in sight. Nate sent us a picture of his new room; his bed was crisply made, corners razor sharp, and quite aesthetically pleasing.

Finally, we worked in one of Nate's favorite sayings with Cody eyeing up the elusive parka—"Sweet Baby Jesus!"

Did You Know?

General George Washington established the Purple Heart Medal during the American Revolution at his Continental Army

Headquarters in Newburgh, New York, August 7, 1782, as the first formal system of recognizing soldiers for individual gallantry. Following the American Revolution, the Purple Heart Medal fell into obscurity but was reestablished by the secretary of war in 1932 at the request of General Douglas MacArthur (USMA 1903), Chief of Staff of the United States Army, as a combat decoration awarded to any American service member who is killed or wounded at the hands of the enemy. Since then, West Point graduates have been killed or wounded in every American conflict leading soldiers in combat. The National Purple Heart Hall of Heroes in New Windsor, New York, founded in 2010, honors those West Point graduates, as well as all other recipients of the Purple Heart Medal. The Purple Heart bears the profile of our founding father, General George Washington.

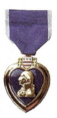

Volume 9: Plebe Parent Weekend! And Now Boxing, March 27, 2018

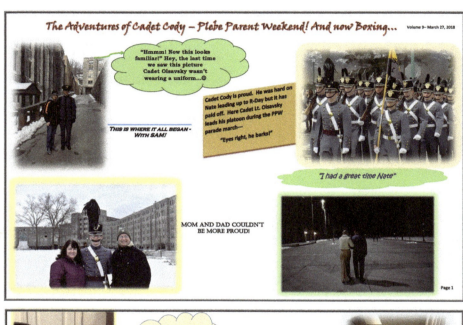

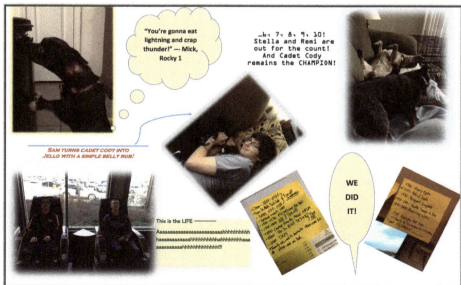

What the Story Is About

Plebe Parent Weekend (PPW) had the look and feel of meet the teacher, show-and-tell, and a school-class play all wrapped up in one. We had the distinguished opportunity to meet Lieutenant Colonel James, Nate's chemistry instructor. Lieutenant Colonel James led a tour of the West Point water treatment facility and provided some information on Lusk Reservoir, located adjacent to Michie Stadium. He quizzed Nate on a Bugle's Notes fact and asked, "Cadet Olsavsky, how many gallons in Lusk Reservoir?"

Nate promptly replied, "Sir, seventy-eight million gallons." Required knowledge for all Plebes.

During this one weekend, Plebes have the academy to themselves and their parents and friends. The upperclassmen are away, and it's all about the Plebes.

Must-sees included the superintendent's welcome, tactical officer's orientation, and barracks open house, academic department open houses, and the uniform factory tour, probably one of our favorites!

During that weekend, Nate was *promoted* to Cadet Lieutenant Olsavsky and led the E-2 platoon in the cadet review parade. What an experience to see Nate wearing a red sash and sword and tar bucket parade hat.

On Saturday night, a banquet was held in the cadet mess hall, a full-dress occasion for all. Following, a formal dress Hop was held at Eisenhower Hall. A very upscale evening!

And after finishing PPW, we welcomed spring break!

What We Really Liked about This Volume

We have an identical picture of Nate and Sam on the ramp adjacent to the admission's building we took when Nate was at West Point for his overnight visit. Now he's wearing a gray uniform—part of the Long Gray Line. It's cool to see the before and after. The parade cadet review picture was edited by Hillary and has the appearance of an oil painting. So nice! I printed a copy and framed it for my brother and Nate's uncle, Mike, who is a postmaster. He has it hanging in his office.

Lastly, yes, Mom and Dad are proud!

Did You Know?

Military working dogs, or MWDs, are trained in various specialties in the Army and other services. There are about 2,500 war dogs in service today, with about 700 serving at any given time overseas. Every MWD is an NCO, noncommissioned officer, in tradition at last. Some say the custom was to prevent handlers from mistreating their dogs; hence, a dog is always one rank higher than its handler.

Volume 10: Up Next Is Sabalauski Air Assault School, May 31, 2018

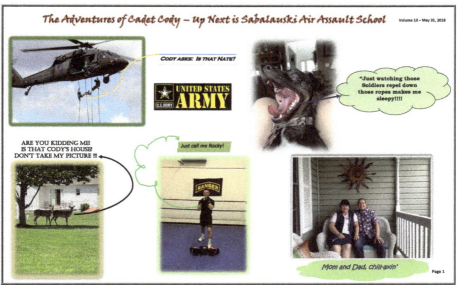

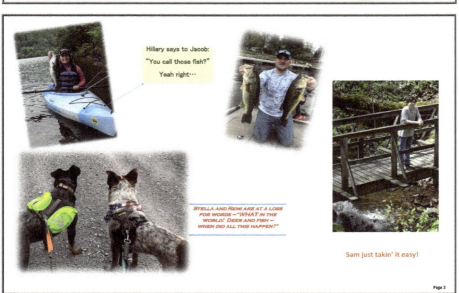

What the Story Is About

Plebe year is coming to a dramatic end, and Nate is anxiously awaiting to hear news of what, if any, air assault (AA) school class he may be attending.

He's in! Group 1, perfect! No downtime between finishing his semester, Plebe year-end TEES and the beginning of AA school. He's excited and we're anxious to see him successfully earn his AA wings.

With air assault completed, Nate now has some free time away from West Point. Home sweet home! And now Nate finally comes clean with what boxing class involved and how he survived. He said he would tell us everything but kept his lips sealed while he was taking boxing class. He didn't want to worry Mom. Cathy was in deep anxiety about boxing. When all was said and done, all for naught!

We spent some time hiking and fishing during Nate's break away from the academy, and as you can see, Hillary and Jacob keep reelin' in the bass! Major League Fishing (MLF) has nothing on them.

What We Really Liked about This Volume

This volume is more about our nonhuman counterparts than anything else. Cody's wide-open, canine-glaring yawn was an unmistakable photo-op moment captured by Sam. Shortly thereafter, two deer were prancing in our backyard. Luckily, Cody was napping and missed out on their entrance. He would have had a field day with those two and been off to the races.

A few MLF size bass caught by Hillary and Jacob were choice add-ins for this edition of Cadet Cody. Remi's patriotic flag neckerchief finished off his and Stella's rearview looking loss for words at the sight of the deer.

Did You Know?

The US flag is not backward. You might think the flag patch on the soldier's uniform looks funny with the stars on the right and stripes on the left, but the official website for the flag of the United

States explains this is because it "gives the effect of the flag flying in the breeze as the wearer moves forward."

The colors: The colors of the flag have important meanings. Red symbolizes hardiness and valor, white symbolizes purity and innocence, and blue represents vigilance, perseverance, and justice.

Volume 11: I'm a Yearling Now and Look What I Can Do, August 22, 2018

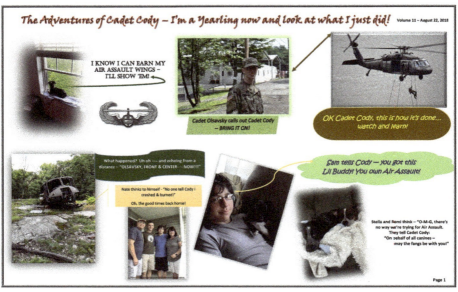

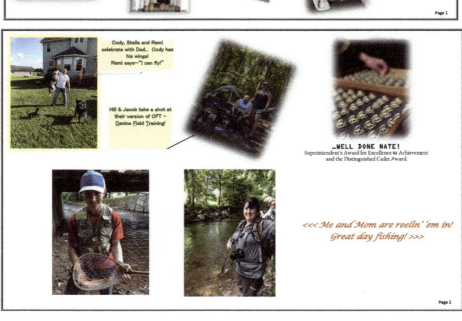

What the Story Is About

Excitement and apprehension. This sums up Nate's emotional capital knowing that he'd be attending the first session of air assault school.

Sabalauski Air Assault School is designed to prepare soldiers for insertion, evacuation, and pathfinding missions that call for the use of multipurpose transportation and assault helicopters. Training is broken into three phases: combat assault, sling load, and rappel. And on graduation day, cadets undergo a twelve-mile rucksack march. Nate loved it!

Nate made his way back home for some much-needed rest, then shortly turned right around to cadet field training (CFT). He took a nasty fall during a reconnaissance exercise and bears the scar on his chin. At least he avoided the black bear sightings at Camp Buckner and the rattlesnake coiled up in one of the barrack bays.

Following CFT, a return back home and some enjoyable hours on one of Pennsylvania's scenic trout streams, Bob's Creek, in Bedford, Pennsylvania. Aunt Susie and Uncle Jim accompanied us on this memorable outing, with Aunt Susie always claiming bragging rights for most fish caught. It's an obsession with her! But to Nate's credit, "check out the palomino rainbow trout I caught!"

What We Really Liked about This Volume

There was so much going on at the end of Nate's Plebe year. Nate earned the Superintendent's Award for Excellence and Achievement and the Distinguished Cadet Award. Well deserved.

Watching Nate repelling from a UH-60 helicopter during air assault school is something that I'll never forget. A memory etched in stone. Those air assault wings are now being proudly worn.

Did You Know?

Excerpts from USCC Cir 351-2, dated May 9, 2017, New Cadet Handbook, Cadet Basic Training 2017, Legends and Traditions of the Corps.

1. How were cadets greeted at West Point in the 1850s? New cadets were greeted by a barrage of buttons fired from a brass candlestick loaded with gunpowder as they reported to their first sergeant for duty.

2. When did the corps stand to arms? In the New York riots against the draft of 1863, word reached West Point that a mob was going to visit and burn the academy. Ball cartridges were issued to the cadets. Pickets of cadets with a field gun at each point were established at the North and South Docks and Gee's Point. No attack was made, however.

3. Who was Pyrene? Cats used to be kept in the old mess to control the mice, and the senior cat on duty was always called Pyrene.

NOTES

PUBLISHED OR BROADCAST sources of information used in this book are cited in the following references/notes as items where text has been utilized to enhance the story theme:

1. *West Point 1915: Eisenhower, Bradley, and the Class the Stars Fell On*, October 17, 2014, by Michael E. Haskew.
2. Army.mil, Carrie McLeroy, Defense Media Activity, December 6, 2016
3. Wikipedia.org, USMA
4. United States Military Academy: 19 Cool Facts, Greg Boudonck, July 26, 2016, part-time-commander.com
5. Wikipedia.org, Army Mules
6. Wikipedia.org, Michie Stadium
7. Fun Facts, West Point Association of Graduates, west-pointaog.org
8. Army.mil, "Military Working Dogs: Guardians of the Night," by Linda Crippen, May 23, 2011
9. "Dogs of War: 23 Facts You Never Knew about Military Working Dogs," Groomsmencentral.com
10. The American Flag, USA.gov
11. Armytimes.com, "Top 5 Duty Stations in the Army," by John Fannin, American Grit, January 18, 2018

12. Onlinecollege.org, "10 Most Prestigious Military Academies in the World"
13. Nationalcenter.org, General Douglas MacArthur's Farewell Speech Given to the Corps of Cadets at West Point, May 12, 1962
14. GoArmywestpoint.com, Washington Establishment quote
15. "Welcome to the United States Military Academy Class of 2021" presentation by Lt. Gen. Robert Caslen, fifty-ninth superintendent of West Point, presented on July 3, 2017
16. The Army, the Army Historical Foundation, 2001, Beaux Arts Edition
17. *Tribune-Review*, Emma Curtis and Nate Smallwood, "Somerset teen enjoys being 'pilot for a day' at 911th Airlift Wing," June 27, 2017
18. West Point Leadership, "Profiles of Courage: Inspirational Profiles of West Point Graduates Who Have Shaped Our World, May 2013, published by Leadership Development Foundation, page 14, "Spotlight"
19. New American Bible, Revised Catholic Edition, Acts of the Apostles, chapter 20, verse 35
20. Army.mil.com, "US Military Academy New Cadet Barracks: Stands for One Its Own" by Joanne Castagna (USACE), May 17, 2017
21. Theculturetrip.com, 12 Cool Facts about the United States Flag
22. 2017 West Point Cemetery Brochure
23. Nasa.gov, "Preparing for the August 2017 Total Solar Eclipse," December 14, 2016
24. History.mil.com, US Army Center of Military History, West Point Museum
25. Military.com, "Army Honors 10th Mountain with 'Pando Commando' Uniforms" by Michael Hoffman, December 4, 2017
26. Army.mil, "The Eggnog Riot" by Carol S. Funck, US Army Heritage and Education Center, December 22, 2010
27. Wikipedia.org, Eggnog Riot

28. "Punching through Barriers: Female Cadets Integrated into Mandatory Boxing at West Point," Association of the United States Army by Maj. Alex Bedard, Maj. Robert "Pete" Peterson, Ray "Coach" Barone, December 16, 2017

29. Pointerview.com, "Alan Alda teaches cadets how to communicate effectively," John Amble, March 8, 2018.

30. Westpointaog.org, The Cadet Uniform Factory-West Point Association of Graduates, "Outfitting the Long Gray Line Since 1878" by Ted Spiegel *West Point Magazine*, spring 2016

31. Code of Federal Regulations, Title 32 Section 578.23, National Defense Service Medal

32. Westpointband.wordpress.com, The Pass in Review, Staff Sergeant Dave Loy Song, May 27, 2014

33. Shea Stadium, Army Athletics, March 6, 2015

34. *Pointer View*, "Scouts Enjoy 56th Annual Camporee," Kathy Eastwood, May 10, 2018

35. *Pointer View*, "Air Assault! From the HLZ!" Cadet David Santos and Cadet McKenzie Bell, June 14, 2018

36. US Department of Defense News, "Chairman Stresses Change, Tradition at West Point Graduation," Jim Garamone (*DoD News*), May 26, 2018

37. *Desert Review*, "US Military Academy West Point names ceremony after hero Captain Scott Pace," Katherine Ramos, October 29, 2018

38. Parks.ny.gov, Walkway Over the Hudson State Historic Park, Parks Recreation and Historic Preservation

39. Pointerview.com, "Building a team, inspiration at Gettysburg," Second Lieutenant Nicholas E. Trux, August 25, 2016

40. Army.mil, "West Point grads get assignments through new branching system," Brandon O'Çonnor, November 18, 2019

41. Wikipedia.org, peridot

42. US Centers for Disease Control (CDC), www.cdc.gov/coronavirus/index.html

43. Army.mil, "Plans in place to safely welcome Class of 2020 back to West Point," Brandon O'Çonnor, May 20, 2020
44. Stripes.com, Stars and Stripes, "Pinks and Greens-inspired uniforms will be issued to soldiers in 2021, Army says" by Christian Lopez, June 12, 2020
45. Pilot Officer John Gillespie Magee: "High Flight" https://www.nationalmuseum.af.mil/Visit/Museum-Exhibits/Fact-Sheets/Display/Article/196844/pilot-officer-john-gillespie-magee-high-flight/
46. www.Westpoint.edu Class of 2021 Crest—West Point

ABOUT THE AUTHOR

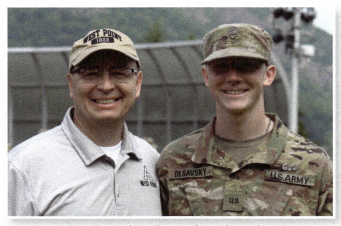

"Joe Olsavsky and Cadet Nathaniel J. Olsavsky—
Sabalauski Air Assault School graduation. June 9, 2018."

JOSEPH E. OLSAVSKY resides in the scenic Laurel Highlands in southwestern Pennsylvania, located fifteen minutes from the Flight 93 National Memorial. Joe and his wife, Cathy, along with their three children, consider their faith and love of family and friends to be most important to them. In the winter of 2017, they welcomed their very first pet to the Olsavsky household: a warm, tiny, fun-loving bundle of canine joy named Cody. Two significant life-changing events also began the year: spinal fusion surgery for Sam, the youngest of their three children, and the countdown to Reception Day (better known as R-Day) at the United States Military Academy at West Point for Nate, their middle child. Writing and publishing a book has been a lifelong dream of Joe's. *The Adventures of Cadet Cody*, his first book, recounts the events leading up to the send-off and goodbye to Nate as he embarks on his future in the US Army.

CPSIA information can be obtained
at www.ICGtesting.com
Printed in the USA
BVHW051707220721
612636BV00021B/1068